Recovering at Home after a Stroke

ALSO BY FLORENCE WEINER

No Apologies: A Guide to Living with a Disability
Help for the Handicapped Child
How to Survive in New York with Children
Peace is You and Me

ALSO BY MATHEW H. M. LEE

Rehabilitation, Music, and Human Well-Being, ed.

ALSO BY FLORENCE WEINER, MATHEW H. M. LEE, AND
HARRIET BELL

Recovering At Home with a Heart Condition

The Howard A. Rusk Institute
of Rehabilitation Medicine

Recovering at Home after a Stroke

A Practical Guide
for You and Your Family

By Florence Weiner,
Mathew H. M. Lee, M.D., F.A.C.P.,
and Harriet Bell, Ph.D.

THE BODY PRESS / PERIGEE

The Client Home-Care Bill of Rights is reprinted by permission of the Foundation for Hospice and Homecare.

The Body Press/Perigee Books
are published by
The Berkley Publishing Group
200 Madison Avenue
New York, NY 10016

Library of Congress Cataloging-in-Publication Data

Weiner, Florence.
    Recovering at home after a stroke : a practical guide for
you and your family / by Florence Weiner, Mathew H. M. Lee, and
Harriet Bell.
        p.   cm.
    At head of title: The Howard A. Rusk Institute of Rehabilitation
Medicine.
    ISBN 0-399-51843-6
    1. Cerebrovascular disease—Patients—Rehabilitation.
2. Cerebrovascular disease—Patients—Home care.   I. Lee,
Mathew H. M.   II. Bell, Harriet.   III. New York University. Rusk
Institute of Rehabilitation Medicine.   IV. Title.
    RC388.5.W44   1994   93-42637   CIP
    616.8'1—dc20

Cover design by Judith Kazdym Leeds
Printed in the United States of America
1   2   3   4   5   6   7   8   9   10

Acknowledgments

The professional excellence and encouragement of the rehabilitation medical staff, the physical therapists, occupational therapists, speech and language pathologists, and psychologists of the Rusk Institute made this book possible.

The insights and recommendations of our professional and consumer advisers made the material more useful.

The wisdom and firsthand experiences of men and women who have had a stroke ultimately shaped this book.

We are indebted to each of them.

Contents

Chapter Four: **A Family Endeavor** 111

• *How Caregiving Family Members Can Help in Recovery*

Chapter Five: **Taking Charge of Your Health** 141

• *The Rusk rehabilitation team gives advice on getting the best medical care; your responsibilities to yourself; and ways to establish a partnership with health-care professionals*

Foreword

Just as exciting as the surgical, pharmaceutical, and other recent advances in medicine is the current trend toward the active participation of human beings in their own care. Three dramatic changes in the perspective of professionals and the general public relate to: (1) the importance of the individual ("the Patient") in the recovery process; (2) the indispensable role of the family and other "caregivers"; and (3) the emphasis on recovering at home with the help of a professionally guided rehabilitation program that achieves its greatest potential *after* the person leaves the hospital.

These developments are particularly significant for the person who has had a stroke. The stroke survivor is no longer a passive recipient but can now be an active participant in a comprehensive rehabilitation program. The results of these changes are exciting—inspiring hope and optimism in people who have had a stroke and in their families.

We all control our own lives by making decisions daily about our diet, exercise, stress levels, our use of drugs, tobacco, and alcohol, as well as through other lifestyle choices. These decisions affect the prevention and treatment of many medical conditions. A stroke is no exception. Although a stroke takes place suddenly, its cause is not from out of nowhere. And when a stroke happens, it doesn't warrant an attitude of doom and resignation that nothing can be done.

In the past, the best medical advice to a person with a stroke may have been simply to rest and hope for a gradual restoration of mobility and other functions. While time is still the great healer, today we know that much more can be accomplished by taking action than by merely lying in bed and waiting for nature to take its course.

Dr. Howard A. Rusk was one of the pioneers in rehabilitation medicine. Only a few decades ago, Dr. Rusk's views were considered radical and perhaps overly optimistic. When he founded the Rusk Institute of Rehabilitation Medicine, he emphasized the importance of establishing a team of physicians and other therapists dedicated to improving the individual's abilities to carry out everyday activities.

In the case of stroke, treatment in the hospital and afterward is often necessary for a variety of cardiovascular, gastrointestinal, urinary, and other related medical conditions. After this initial treatment, the emphasis is on rehabilitation—training and empowering the person to return to their everyday routine, both at home and, if possible, at work. And with the continuing trend toward shorter hospital stays for everyone, the emphasis on recovery at home is even more vital to the person with a stroke.

Cardiovascular problems, cancer, and stroke are three of the most common medical conditions affecting people today. Almost everyone knows about the dramatic new techniques in preventing and treating heart attacks and other cardiovascular conditions, and cancer. But most people know very little about stroke.

A stroke is the disruption of the blood supply to or within the brain. When the blood supply is cut off, the brain does not receive the oxygen and nutrients it needs, and the result is damage to the brain cells. If the cells are damaged or die from lack of oxygen, the body functions controlled by these brain cells are affected.

Every year approximately half a million Americans have a stroke. More than two million people in this country have had one or more strokes. Stroke is one of the most common causes of physical disability. In fact, stroke is usually the most common diagnosis found in medical rehabilitation programs. Although stroke is often considered a disease of the elderly, and the incidence of stroke does increase with age, one-quarter of all strokes occur in people *under* the age of sixty.

A person who has had heart-bypass surgery can return to work in a few weeks. A person who has had a heart attack is able to talk vigorously about its causes and treatment to relatives, friends, and coworkers. But this is less likely to be the case with a stroke. A person who has had a stroke is more likely to have problems with speech, vision, and movement, as well as other medical complications. The rehabilitation of a stroke survivor often requires very hard work over a period of months or years.

When I first started working with Dr. Rusk, rehabilitation medicine was a new term. I remember how often Dr. Rusk reminded me to think of medical rehabilitation as the third phase of medicine, following preventive medicine and curative medicine and surgery. Today, I look at medical rehabilitation as a dynamic process. I see that rehabilitation concepts and procedures start at the earliest possible moment following an acute illness or injury and permeate every aspect of the subsequent treatment.

Much of Dr. Rusk's early work was with people with severe disabilities: soldiers who were amputees, polio survivors who lived in iron lungs, and young people who had been in automobile or sports accidents that resulted in motor and sensory paralysis. Our work with thousands of people with these disabilities has helped in the development of therapeutic techniques and services for people with strokes. The Rusk Institute's work with aphasia, physical, occupational, and recreational therapies, and psychological and vocational counseling is the basis for much of this book.

Hundreds of specialized physicians and other therapists have trained at the Rusk Institute. Of particular relevance to a person who has had a stroke is the array of professionals who are *not* physicians—the nurses, physical, occupational, and recreational therapists, speech and language pathologists, psychologists, social workers, dietitians, and others.

Nowadays, most hospitals have an early-discharge policy, so that people are likely to return home "quicker and sicker." Families often have acute nursing-care responsibilities for loved ones who only days before were in a professionally staffed and fully equipped intensive-care unit. In these cases, families should be encouraged to join in physical, occupational, and speech-therapy sessions *during* the hospital stay in order to have a better understanding of how to continue this valuable work at home. At Rusk, we believe that nothing replaces the skill of trusted and caring professionals. But we also consider family members and other caregiving friends and helpers as valuable partners on the rehabilitation team. We acknowledge the healing power that comes from their love, hard work, and compassionate concern.

After several decades as a rehabilitation physician, I continue to be touched and gratified when I see the bonding of a family around the stroke survivor, especially when the work of recovery is viewed as a positive challenge. Instead of pulling away and disintegrating, the family and friends who join the rehabilitation team become partners in miracles.

As the Medical Director of the Rusk Institute of Rehabilitation Medicine, I am keenly aware of the imminent neurological and other medical breakthroughs that will help prevent stroke, reduce the likelihood of recurrent strokes, and dramatically reduce the effects of stroke within the next decade. As a physiatrist, I have seen the remarkable advances in all aspects of rehabilitative medicine.

Another, more subtle, breakthrough in the medical community is one in attitude, signaled by the diminishing use of the word "patient." The Latin origin of this word is "to suffer." The word evolved to mean a person who *receives* medical attention, care, or treatment. But today, the person with a medical problem is an active participant in their healing process and involved in all decision making. That's why you will not find the word "patient" anywhere in the pages that follow. We also try to avoid technical and professional jargon, even though you're probably already aware of some of the more commonly used medical terms, like IV (short for intravenous).

This is not a medical reference book. It is a self-help guide for a person who has survived a stroke and for family members and others on the rehabilitation team. The authors' overall philosophy is motivated by the desire to provide a book that is useful and easily understood in its suggestions, advice, and strategies. And most important, we hope to be as supportive and empowering to you as you will allow us to be.

Dr. Howard A. Rusk touched the lives of all three authors. I was trained in rehabilitation medicine by Dr. Rusk. Florence Weiner's sister had her rehabilitation training at the Rusk Institute following an accident. Dr. Bell lived for twenty-five years in the Howard A. Rusk Respiratory Unit of Goldwater Memorial Hospital and now lives in the community.

The purpose of this book is to encourage you to become actively involved in your recovery process so that you may reach your maximum level of independence. We look forward to hearing if we have helped you succeed.

Mathew H. M. Lee, M.D., F.A.C.P.
Medical Director
Rusk Institute of Rehabilitation Medicine
New York University Medical Center
New York, New York

Introduction

"Even if you are optimistic by nature, having a stroke comes as a crushing blow. You wonder why this happened to you and what your life will be like," says Howard Feinstein, who had a stroke at age fifty-two—two and a half years ago. "Once you know you are going to live, having a stroke is no different than any other life-altering crisis you face. The main point is it happened, and there's not too much you can do about that. What you can do is carry on the long, slow, and hard fight—and not quit—so you can go forward and beyond it." Further, he says, "You are entitled to your hurts, anger, and feelings of loss for things that are different, and the right to ask for the help you need."

"A stroke changes the way you live your life, but it doesn't change wanting to have a life. Once you figure out what you need and want and who can help you get it, you have a chance to put the pieces back together to rebuild your life," Feinstein asserts.

This book focuses on the personal side of living after a stroke, rather than on the medical aspects of recovery. It attempts to deal with some of the difficulties you may encounter and provides strategies, advice, and suggested questions for your doctor, nurses, physical therapists, speech therapists, occupational therapists, and social workers. It also helps you find ways to back up the valuable work of these rehabilitation professionals in the context of your own home. It's meant to reach you when you are most concerned about how you will be able to function, the strains your care may have on your family, and what the quality of life will be for you and your family.

Chances are that if you are reading this book, you are a close family member or friend of someone who has had a stroke and you want to know where to find home health-care services, information, products—the essentials for practical and meaningful support in your caregiving role. Or you yourself may have sustained a stroke and would like recommendations from professionals on how to make life work again, as well as firsthand advice from men and women with experiences similar to yours.

Understandably, you and your family may not have had a chance to think about your recovery at home while you were still in a hospital bed or in the early stages of your rehabilitation. So let this book be your guide to the positive challenges that lie ahead through the entire spectrum of the healing process and to the sources of support you may call upon.

It's comforting to know that whatever you want to accomplish doesn't have to be done all at once or by yourself. You can call upon members of your family, friends, and/or someone you employ to assist you as well as health-care professionals, who can make the work less arduous.

This book will point you in the direction of dozens of new allies and helpers, ranging from your doctor to nurses, physical therapists and speech therapists, occupational therapists, dietitians, social workers, psychologists and psychiatrists, along with new friends that you and your family can meet at stroke support groups. It will also lead you to discover some of the untapped possibilities among your own existing support system of family and friends. You and your family can focus on different chapters in this book as your needs change and as you move from one recovery stage to the next.

Initially, your family will want to know which questions to ask before you leave the hospital. So, for example, you'll find specific questions to ask the nurse about your care at home, such as arranging your home for greater self-sufficiency and safety and which medical supplies to have on hand. You, your family, and the people who work with you will want to know the results of the evaluations made by your doctor, nurses, and the other professionals who are involved regarding your present ability to balance while sitting and standing, to move about, to see, and to sense hot, cold, sharp, and soft, so that you will not hurt yourself.

While recovering, you will need to know about scheduling your medications; whether to double the dosage the next time if you forget to take a dose; the possible reactions to the medications; and which signs and symptoms must be reported to your doctor. You, your family, and people with whom you work or spend time away from home should know the indications of an emergency, the steps to take should an emergency occur, and how to get immediate medical help. Since most office visits with your doctor and other health professionals are relatively brief, you may want to know how to make the most of the time spent together and your rights as a medical consumer.

In the book's special-resource section, you'll find games and computer software recommended by speech therapists to strengthen your communication skills. It also includes information about where to buy or rent a wheelchair, a bath or shower chair, and useful products for greater independence in eating, bathing, dressing, communicating, hearing, reading, and driving. Also described are community organizations that provide services to ease the transition from hospital to home, from home to work, or doing the other things that matter to you.

* * *

Start reading this book at the point where you now are in your recovery. Family members can make notes in the margins. Consider making several copies of the charts so that you can use them for as long as you like.

The following chapter summaries can serve as a guide:

Chapter One: Leaving the Hospital Here is the kind of information you and your family will want to gather from the hospital staff. It includes specific questions to ask the doctors, the nurses, the physical therapists, the occupational therapists, and the speech therapists about your care at home. The social workers and hospital discharge planners will direct the family to the appropriate home-care services and professional visits and explain the insurance coverage for these services.

Chapter Two: Recovering at Home From the staff of the Rusk Institute you find practical advice on how to plan your day and create an informal daily schedule. Here are suggested ways to arrange your bedroom, bathroom, and kitchen so that clothes and utensils are within easy reach; plus tips on living with the use of one hand in a two-handed world. A chart provides suggestions on how-to create your own individual schedule, with space to record your blood pressure, medications, and any comments you want to share with your doctor.

Chapter Three: Being Safe Physical therapists and occupational therapists provide a room-by-room checklist for preventing home accidents, point out the most common accident sites, and offer suggestions for creating a barrier-free environment. The everyday role of the family in averting and handling emergencies is discussed. Also covered are the specific steps to take in an emergency, should one occur, and guidelines to determine the warning signs of a recurrence of a stroke.

Chapter Four: A Family Endeavor Families share their experiences and offer advice on how to care for a family member after a stroke—without hindering self-direction, or forfeiting lives of their own. Speech and cognition therapists suggest ways to enhance communication and memory skills in the home. Included are strategies for all family members to help them conserve their energy. You also will find a description of home-care services and their costs, plus suggestions for locating and training a personal-care aide—without going through an agency. Also discussed in this chapter is how to establish the kind of partnership with home-care professionals that can help maintain and enhance your equality, dignity, and independence.

Chapter Five: Taking Charge of Your Health The Rusk Institute rehabilitation medical team offers practical advice on how to find the best medical care and discusses the medical specialists who treat stroke. You will also discover new ways to establish a sound partnership with your doctor. Here are dozens of suggested questions to ask your doctor about your medical condition, medications, and the signs and symptoms that need to be reported. There is a chart to be used as a medication reminder, with spaces to record each dose.

Chapter Six: Lifelong Learning Here are tips and strategies from the Rusk Institute's physical, occupational, and speech therapists on implementing their valuable work at home. Occupational therapists and psychologists offer guidelines on how to enhance memory and how to use a computer, games, and other devices. Also discussed is how to set short-term goals, and the type of professionals who can help you maintain your program. Practical techniques are outlined to help you cope with depression, stress, and the other emotional reactions to stroke. The chapter tells how other men and women who have had a stroke can help strengthen you. Suggestions for incorporating regular, safe exercise into your routine, and how to prepare easy-to-eat nutritious meals are provided here. There's also a chart to support your efforts to quit smoking, plus sensitive, sensible reassurance and helpful information about intimacy.

Chapter Seven: Information, Services, and Products Sources for locating the home-care services in your community and other kinds of support for caregiving families are provided, as well as suggestions for finding physical therapists, occupational therapists, speech pathologists, social workers, and other professional services, including psychological counseling and support groups. Included are a section on where to buy, rent, or borrow useful products to help you in the recovery process; a selection of books about stroke, blood pressure, diabetes, and other medical subjects, plus cookbooks and books about a mind/body approach to healing; and pertinent newsletters and audiotapes.

Each chapter ends with a brief interview with a person who is currently recovering after a stroke, or whose close family member is recovering after a stroke. To protect their privacy, some of the interviewees are identified by pseudonyms.

Here are some suggestions on how best to use this book:

- Purchase a school notebook or loose-leaf binder and arrange it as if it were a calendar, or by subject, or in any way that makes it easiest to use according to your own personal preferences.
- Every time you come across a specific item that seems especially valuable to you, enter the page number and topic in your notebook.
- Begin this book by looking on page 260, where you will find a place to keep the telephone numbers of your doctor, personal-care attendants, people at the hospital who can answer your questions once you are home, your insurance policy numbers, and numbers

to call in an emergency. Make a copy for your notebook or fill it in directly onto the page in this book;
flag it with a Post-It, tab, or paper clip so you may
find the page again quickly.

- You may want to use a binder or folder to save bills
and organize them into two categories: "PAID" and
"UNPAID." Be sure to keep receipts from any health-
care-related purchases, contracts from home-care
agencies and suppliers, pertinent letters, and whatever else is worthwhile saving for your own records
or for insurance and tax purposes.

As this book points you to the facts and resources you
seek for your recovery process, you will find that some of
the questions are simple and easy to have answered. But if
a question is relevant to you and you can't find the answer,
don't ignore it and give up; keep on trying until you get the
information you need.

This book would not be possible without the interviews
with many experts on the subject of stroke, especially the
professionals at the Rusk Institute of Rehabilitation Medicine, and at other hospitals, medical facilities, and organizations. Most important, however, were the one-on-one
meetings and telephone conversations with dozens of
people who have had a stroke. We thank you for your help
and inspiration.

Chapter One

Leaving the Hospital

What lies behind us and what lies before us are tiny matters compared to what lies within us.
—RALPH WALDO EMERSON

MAKING THE TRANSITION FROM HOSPITAL TO HOME: ADVICE FROM MEN AND WOMEN WHO HAVE HAD A STROKE

"When I was about to leave the hospital, if someone who had had a stroke said to me: 'Listen, it's hard work recovering from a stroke, but I've done it, and so can you,' I would have been a lot less frightened," says Natalie DiMico, fifty-three, who had a stroke two years ago.

"I was grateful to be alive, but at first I couldn't do the things I once took for granted. My doctor, the nurses, physical therapists, occupational therapists, and speech therapists weren't going home with me, and I was scared about how I would manage, and so was my husband."

Families agree that making the transition from hospital to home after a stroke is an unnerving experience. It takes several people—whether family members or friends—to gather the information from the hospital staff, arrange for a visiting nurse, a personal-care aide, and for physical, occupational, and speech therapy; obtain prescriptions, a written hospital discharge plan, and your medical records. Also, your family will want to prepare for your homecoming, arranging the bedroom, bathroom, and kitchen—perhaps installing bars in the bathtub and shower or a ramp over a step—so that you will have the greatest measure of accessibility, safety, and self-sufficiency.

After a stroke, most people are discharged from the hospital within ten days, while others stay longer or transfer to a rehabilitation center. Whether you are in the hospital for only a matter of days or for several weeks, you and your family have ample opportunity to talk with your doctor, the nurses, and physical, occupational, and speech therapists about their evaluation of what you can do on your own and what activities may require assistance. With

these known guidelines, family members and other
helpers can support you in reaching the highest level of
self-sufficiency possible, and they are less likely to either
overprotect or push you.

When families have an idea of the nursing care and
other therapies required and know what costs are *not*
covered by insurance, they then can make the necessary
financial plans. As they learn more about what to expect
in the actual experience of their new daily routine, they
can address some basic concerns. How may responsibilities be shared among family members? Personal
care, shopping, preparing and serving meals, and provid-
ing transportation should be handled so that the primary
caregiver does not become overwhelmed. Paid assistance
may be needed to augment what the primary caregiver
and others in the family can offer. Will the family's financial resources be sufficient for personal care and household expenses? Are modifications to the home needed to
make it accessible and safe? If you live alone or caregiving
family members live at a distance, which support services
must you have to continue living in your home?

Families who have had similar experiences offer these
suggestions and recommendations about what you can
do when leaving the hospital:

While in the hospital, choose an advocate. A family
member or close friend can be your representative or
"advocate." The person should sit in on all discussions
with your doctor, the nurses, physical, occupational, and
speech therapists, and social workers. Your representative can compose questions beforehand and have a combination notebook/datebook available to take down the
answers to your questions, as well as other pertinent
notes. Another section in the notebook could be set aside
for the names and telephone numbers of your doctor,
therapists, the home-care agency, personal-care aide, and
other frequently used phone numbers. You also want to

have the telephone numbers and extensions of staff members who said they would answer questions after you leave the hospital. In a datebook, keep a record of the dates and times of future doctor, therapy, and other appointments.

Compile a list of specific questions for the person on staff who is most likely to be able to answer the questions. You and your family will want to draw from each professional who has had a role in your hospital care as much information as you need. Your doctor should be able to answer questions about your stroke, the effect it has had on you, and address your concerns about the future as well. Suggested questions for you to ask the doctors may be found on page 149.

The nurses can answer questions about the care needed at home, how to schedule medications, and the specialty items that you may need to have on hand. Physical therapists can demonstrate the prescribed exercises. In addition, be sure to get *written instructions* for you, your family, and others who will assist you while doing the exercises and in maintaining the proper positions for body alignment while sitting, standing, or lying in bed. They and the occupational therapists can teach family members and other helpers how to assist you between sessions in developing strategies for use in everyday tasks. Occupational therapists impart beneficial techniques for participating in recreational activities as well as dealing with job training. Speech therapists can teach you techniques to stimulate memory and instruct you and your family in ways to improve and enhance communications at home. Suggested questions for the nurses and physical, occupational, and speech therapists may be found throughout this chapter.

Try not to be intimidated or feel that you are bothering someone when you ask for help. Family members need to remember: go slowly, be courteous and assertive, and focus on getting the information you want. If something is unclear to you, ask again, or ask someone else until you understand it. Bring up questions and concerns that are important to you, even if they haven't been covered by the staff.

Social workers are responsible for helping families make the transition from the hospital to home. If family members want arrangements made for home-nursing visits and physical, occupational, and speech therapy, they should initiate the appointment with the social-work department, rather than waiting for them to call the family. Discuss the home care prescribed by your doctor. Either the social worker or your own insurance representative can tell you whether your insurance plan will cover it. There may be a limit to the number of visits that are fully covered, or you may be responsible for partial payments.

Most hospitals have at least one social worker or other staff member who can arrange the home-care nursing and therapy prescribed by your doctor through their own agency or an affiliate. This office usually provides prescribed assistive devices, such as a cane, a walker, or a wheelchair. You are under no obligation to take the home-care services or assistive devices provided by the hospital planning office. In fact, arrangements may *not* be made for any services, therapists, or assistive devices by the hospital planning office without the permission of a family.

Many families make their own arrangements for home-nursing care, physical and speech therapy, and assistive devices. If the family so chooses, remember to make sure that the home-care agency you opt for is approved by your insurance company so that you will be appropriately reimbursed. If a personal-care aide is needed for an extended period of time, you may prefer to make these arrangements on your own. For more information about finding and training a personal-care aide, see page 130.

If a wheelchair, walker, or cane is expected to be used for only a short period of time after the hospital, these items may be rented or borrowed rather than purchased. Of course, you will need them in time for leaving the hospital, so make the necessary arrangements in advance. Insurance may not reimburse you for *rental* costs incurred for a wheelchair or walker but often will cover the item if it is purchased. See page 232 for a list of sources that rent medical equipment, along with the organizations that have equipment for loan.

You are entitled to a written hospital discharge plan before leaving the hospital. If you are not given a written discharge plan, your family will need to ask for one. Hospital discharge plans should include detailed instructions about your medications, diet, home-nursing care, and visits from physical, occupational, and speech therapists. If anything on the discharge plan is unclear, it should be explained to the family by a nurse or social worker.

Prescriptions are needed for medications. Either your doctor or the nurse will give a family member the prescriptions for your medication. A family member may want to do some comparison shopping before filling a prescription simply by phoning several pharmacies in the neighborhood. When you give the pharmacist the name of the medication, the dosage amount, and number of tablets, you may find that prices can vary greatly.

Prescriptions are needed for physical therapy, speech therapy, occupational therapy, home-nursing visits, and assistive devices. Therapists, medical-supply stores, and home-care agencies require a prescription for services and assistive devices. To be reimbursed by insurance for home care and therapy, the services must be covered by your plan and be accompanied by a prescription from your doctor.

A patient advocate is on the staff of most hospitals. Increasingly, hospitals have patient advocates who can be helpful in answering the family's questions or in addressing your complaints. If they cannot answer the questions, they will direct you to the person who can.

Ask how to obtain a copy of your medical records. Your doctor, the social worker, or patient advocate should be able to tell the family how to obtain a copy of your medical records from the hospital. Ask the doctor who has been treating you in the hospital to send a complete report of your hospitalization to each of your other doctors.

You can continue to get information and recommendations after you have been discharged from the hospital. At all stages of your recovery you have an opportunity for an ongoing relationship with your doctor and therapists. As new questions and concerns arise, you may feel free to consult them at home and in their offices for the answers you need and to learn the purpose of their recommendations. It may be easier to evaluate and obtain maximum benefit from the services of the health-care professionals with whom you work if you think of yourself as a "medical consumer." For more about your rights on this subject, see page 136.

SPECIFIC QUESTIONS THE NURSING STAFF CAN ANSWER

Integral to nursing care is teaching you to be more confident about caring for yourself. Nurses also give instructions to caregiving family members so that they know the care that will be most beneficial for you. But since relatively few days are spent in the hospital, the nursing staff doesn't have much time to teach you and your family about your specific needs at home. While you're in the hospital, you and your family should try to be as alert as possible to what you can learn about everyday activities. It may be difficult, but the last few days in the hospital are the most important time to practice—as well as you can—sitting up and maintaining your balance, transferring from the bed to a chair or wheelchair, dressing, eating, bathing, and doing exercises. At home, these activities will continue with a family member or other helper assisting you.

Many families decide to have several home-nursing visits when the person who has had the stroke is first discharged from the hospital. Even if the nursing services are not prescribed or reimbursable by their insurance plan, families generally find that a visit from a home-care nurse is worth the cost. Not only do these nurses evaluate the progress of recovery and report their recommendations to the doctor, they are also an excellent source of information about local community services, reliable vendors, and other professionals. Families find that home-care nursing is especially valuable if the family member who has had the stroke is elderly, and also has arthritis, high blood pressure, or heart or respiratory conditions that require special medical procedures, such as giving injections and monitoring blood pressure and pulse. Most important, however, is the fact that most families find that arranging for one or several visits from a home-care nurse adds immeasurably to their confidence: the experiences can provide the reassurance they need to manage on their own. (For more about home nursing care, see Chapter Two, "Recovering at Home," page 49.)

Here are some suggested questions the family may want to ask the hospital nursing staff or a visiting nurse.

- Are there detailed instructions on medications, diet, physical therapy, speech therapy, and occupational therapy in the hospital discharge plan? Are there instructions that the primary caregiver needs to have explained? Don't be shy about asking.

- What should the primary family caregiver and other helpers know about home care, including the scheduling of medications, monitoring pulse and blood pressure, incontinence, depression, disorientation? Are there side effects from the medications that need to be reported to the doctor?
- What do the family caregivers and other helpers need to know about the purpose and scheduling of each of the medications? Are there potentially serious side effects from the medications that we should be aware of?
- Should blood pressure be taken at home? If so, how often? Is there anything else that we should monitor at home and record for the visiting nurse, physical therapist, or doctor?
- What are the signs and symptoms the family and other helpers need to recognize that may indicate an emergency?
- What medical supplies or other equipment are needed for home care?
- Is there anyone on the nursing staff who can answer questions over the phone after the family member has left the hospital? If so, write down their name(s) and telephone number(s). See page 260 for sample phone list. At hospitals and other larger medical facilities, it's very important to get the specific telephone extension numbers or direct dial numbers.

SPECIFIC QUESTIONS FOR PHYSICAL THERAPISTS

The goals of physical therapy are to restore and/or achieve the optimal movement and function necessary for daily living. Your own personal goals for your therapy are equally important. Before leaving the hospital, you and your family will want to learn the results of the physical therapist's evaluation which determines the strength of your muscles, legs, and trunk, your ability to move your arms and legs, and your sense of balance and coordination. Based on this information, physical therapists plan a treatment program geared to meet your individual needs, goals, abilities, and lifestyle.

The treatment offered by physical therapists may include mobilizing stiff joints and tissue, exercise, stretching, and walking. Family members will continue the valuable work between sessions, learning to assist you without harming themselves as they handle a wheelchair, lift you, and help you move. Physical therapists give out written instructions for the exercises, along with illustrations, and can demonstrate for family members and other helpers the proper way to supervise and assist you. Some families bring a video camera to physical-therapy sessions as a teaching tool and to record progress. Your video camera includes sound, so ask the therapist to provide a voice commentary or instructions.

After the hospital, physical therapy continues at home and then in office visits. In areas where there is a shortage of physical therapists who make home visits, it is often possible for the home-care nurse to supervise the exercises.

Here are some questions families commonly ask physical therapists.

- What types of exercises should be done at home? How often during the day should these exercises be done? How long should each exercise session last?
- Is physical therapy prescribed? Are there instructions in my written hospital discharge plan that need to be explained?
- Other than physical therapy, which activities would I benefit from? Are there activities I should avoid?

- Is there a physical therapy staff member who will
  answer my questions after I leave the hospital? If so,
  write down their name(s), telephone number(s), and
  extension(s).

SPECIFIC QUESTIONS FOR OCCUPATIONAL THERAPISTS

Most people are unaware of what occupational therapists
do until they work with one after an illness or accident.
Occupational therapy encompasses all aspects of everyday living, whether recreational or pertaining to career
and job training. Occupational therapists help people regain the muscular coordination necessary to perform
such basic activities as dressing, bathing, and personal
care. If there is paralysis on one side, occupational therapists teach ways to dress using the sounder side of the
body and may recommend the clothing styles that are
easiest to maneuver.

Occupational therapists also teach individuals and
their families how to use a wheelchair, how to transfer
safely from one place to another, and will recommend
assistive devices that can make the move back home easier and safer.

Here are suggested questions for the occupational therapy staff:

- What exercises or activities should be done at home
  and how often?
- Is occupational therapy prescribed? Are there instructions in my written hospital discharge plan
  about therapy or equipment that need to be explained?
- Has an occupational therapy evaluation been made?

What can you tell me and my family about it? Is there assistive equipment I should have for daily activities? Can you recommend stores in my community where I can purchase the assistive equipment I need?

- Is there an occupational therapy staff member who will answer my questions after I leave the hospital? (If so, make a note of his or her name, telephone number, and extension.)

(If you are interested in finding an occupational therapist, see page 222.)

SPECIFIC QUESTIONS FOR SPEECH THERAPISTS

Speech/language pathologists help people communicate, and that involves far more than speech alone. Whether the stroke is on the left side of the brain, the right side, or in deeper structures, it can alter the ability to comprehend and express information. The stroke may affect listening, attention, remembering what was heard or seen, pronouncing sounds, visual perception, reading, recalling words, forming ideas into spoken messages, spelling, writing, and computing numbers.

One person may experience few of these changes, while another may find many affected. Regardless of the type of communication change, therapists can evaluate how the stroke has disrupted a person's ability to communicate and begin to work on building and strengthening communication skills and developing new ones.

Speech/language pathologists offer guidelines to the entire family on how to encourage language in "teachable moments" that take place naturally throughout a typical day.

Here are suggested questions for the speech therapists:

- Has speech therapy been prescribed? Are there instructions in my written hospital discharge plan that need to be explained?
- Are there exercises or other instructions I should have before continuing speech therapy? What information does my family need?
- Has an evaluation been made? What can you tell me and my family about it?
- Is there a speech therapy staff member who will answer my questions after I leave the hospital? If so, write down his or her name, telephone number, and extension.

(If you are interested in finding a speech/language pathologist, see page 222. Speech and language information and materials are on page 236.)

THE SOCIAL WORK DEPARTMENT: HOSPITAL DISCHARGE PLANNERS AND THEIR SERVICES

Almost every hospital has at least one discharge planner, while others may have a staff of many social workers or nurses. Hospitals vary in their discharge procedures. Since most discharge offices are understaffed and frequently a large number of people leave the hospital at one time, hospital discharge planners do not automatically see everyone. In fact, it's a good idea for you or a family member to call in advance for an appointment, rather than waiting until just prior to being discharged. This is especially important if your doctor orders home-nursing care and you want the hospital discharge planner to arrange it for you.

A social worker or hospital discharge planner can usually order home-nursing care and arrange for physical therapy, speech therapy, and medical equipment and services that have been prescribed by the doctor. However, services and equipment offered by them may be obtained independently by you. Although arrangements for home-care nursing and physical therapy made for you by a discharge planner admittedly are convenient, they may allow you and your family less opportunity to actively participate in the selection process.

For example, you and a family member may decide to interview and hire a personal-care aide, either before entering the hospital for care when you return home or after you are already home. Increasingly, many families decide to have a personal-care aide on a part-time basis—especially if a family member is elderly or has had surgery. For more information about the responsibilities of a personal-care aide and finding one, see page 132.

A nurse or a physical therapist prescribed by your doctor must come from a home-care agency approved by your insurance.

In addition, social workers and psychologists may provide psychological counseling to individuals and families and can recommend sources for additional counseling if needed.

SPECIFIC QUESTIONS FOR SOCIAL WORKERS

- Are all the instructions in my discharge plan complete? Do they include a list of restricted activities, an exercise plan, a diet, and prescribed home-nursing care and physical therapy?
- If we want to make our own arrangements for a

personal-care aide, can you recommend several home-care agencies or other appropriate community resources to consult?

- Will a nurse, physical therapist, and/or speech therapist come to my home? For what length of time? Can you explain my insurance coverage for the prescribed home care?
- Does a stroke support group meet at this hospital? If not, can you suggest a resource that may provide one in or near my community?

CHECKING YOUR HOSPITAL BILL

Before leaving the hospital, you are entitled to a full explanation of your hospital bill. If there are questions about the charges, a family member should make an appointment with the billing office to review the bill.

Two outside organizations that can help you understand your itemized bills are the People's Medical Society and the American Association of Retired Persons.

- The People's Medical Society, 462 Walnut Street, Allentown, PA 18102, 1-800-624-8773, will send you a free fact sheet about decoding your hospital bill and advise you about what to do if you have been overcharged. They will also send a fact sheet on filing a complaint. This consumer health advocacy organization recommends the following when you suspect an error or question a charge on a bill:

    - Request an itemized bill. Contact your insurance company and request an audit of your account. Ask for a Utilization Review. If you're a Medicare recipient, contact your nearest Social Security Administration office.

- Inform the hospital when you have *not* received a treatment or service for which you were charged.
- If you have been charged for services you have *not* received and the hospital threatens you with legal action directly or through a collection agency for nonpayment, contact your state's Consumer Protection Agency.
- If you are still unable to resolve your problem, you may want to consider retaining legal counsel.

- The American Association of Retired Persons, 601 E Street, NW, Washington, DC 20049, 202-434-2277, provides free help in deciphering bills and dealing with insurers. More than thirty-two million people are AARP members. To join, you only have to be fifty years of age or older; you can be working or retired. To learn more about this organization's informational and referral services, as well as discounts for members, see page 227.

A Checklist for the Family

On your last day in the hospital, or shortly after you return home, you and your family should review the materials provided by the various medical professionals and make sure that:

- most of your questions have been answered by your doctor, the nurses, therapists—physical, speech, and occupational—social worker, and dietitian.
- the family has been given a written discharge plan

that lists your medications with complete instructions, your recommended diet and exercise plan, the
prescribed home-nursing services, physical-therapy
program, and list of restricted activities.

• the nurses have informed you of the medical supplies
and items to have on hand for your comfort and
safety, such as a bathtub chair, a hand-held showerhead, and special eating utensils. Many drugstores
and home health-care supply stores stock the items
you need or can order them for you.

• the hospital dietitian has made recommendations
about food preparation and any restrictions in your
diet. If you are experiencing difficulty swallowing or
chewing, the dietitians may be able to recommend
nutritional supplements and ways to prepare food
that will make the process of ingestion easier and
more pleasurable. For more about nutritional needs
and special eating utensils for people who have experienced a stroke, see page 233. For a description of a
nutritionist's services and how to locate one in your
community, see page 222.

• prescriptions for medications, home-care services,
physical therapy, speech therapy, occupational therapy, and any necessary assistive devices—such as a
walker, cane, or wheelchair—have been given to you.

• the family has met with the social worker/discharge
planner and understands the home-care services
available to you, the home-care services prescribed,
and the extent of your insurance coverage. Permission has been given for arrangements to be made by
the discharge planner for a nurse, physical therapist,
or other home-care service, or you have decided to
make your own arrangements.

• you have checked all the charges on the hospital bill
and, if there is an error, it has been adjusted.

• you have requested a complete copy of your hospital
record.

- you know when your next appointment will be with your doctor.
- the family has the names, telephone numbers, and extensions of the hospital staff members who have agreed to answer your questions after you leave the hospital.

Dr. Richard Nelson*, Anesthesiologist and Director of an Ambulatory Surgery Unit

I would say it's true of most physicians that they think "These things don't happen to us; they happen to other people." Logically, we know that we are not exempt from these things and that there are bound to be a number of physicians who get various diseases; but mostly we sort of feel that these things don't happen to us, and when they do occur, we feel it as a far greater shock.

My situation started with a few days of symptoms of a flu-like illness. I realized that I wasn't getting better, my physician was going out of town, so I went into the hospital. The neurological symptoms actually evolved as I was sitting in the emergency room. So I was in the best possible place for such a thing to occur. I was admitted to the hospital for evaluation—and stayed there for about a week—and then spent about two weeks in a rehabilitation center.

I was very, very lucky in that my motor involvement was on a very moderate scale. I have a loss of sensation on the right side of my body, which is getting better; and some very mild motor involvement of the muscles, but I can walk without any problems. I have some loss of fine motor control in my right hand, which is my dominant hand, but I am back at work, even starting IVs in babies. I went through various therapies for about a year before coming back to work.

Apart from going into the hospital for therapy, I had some eye-muscle problems. I went to the local institute of optometry here. I really could fend for myself, unlike people with major motor problems. I did a year of exercising, so the prism glasses usually prescribed played a rela-

* This is a pseudonym.

46

tively minor role for me at first. I struggled for eight or nine months to do the eye therapy, rather than depend on the prism glasses for sight correction. At the institute they suggested that I do the assorted exercises first. The people there were topnotch professionals who were very helpful and very good—innovative and supportive. I was more than impressed.

> "After the stroke, I felt I had two options: I could either lie down and say, 'Well, it's happened, I'm a goner.' Or I could fight like hell to get back what I could."

After the stroke, I felt I had two options: I could either lie down and say, "Well, it's happened, I'm a goner." Or I could fight like hell to get back what I could. I still have some residual problems with the right side and with the eye; I can't drive without prism glasses, otherwise I have double vision. But with the prism glasses, I'm fine. After all, I've gone back to work within the year of having the stroke. So my advice would be to someone else who's had a stroke: "Fight like hell. The doctors can do so much, the nurses can do so much, and then what's left is up to you and the Almighty. And what He can do, you don't know either."

Chapter Two

Recovering at Home

Healing is a matter of time, but it is sometimes also a matter of opportunity.

—HIPPOCRATES

Coming Home

As difficult an experience as hospitalization is, most people can see its purpose and beneficial results. After a stroke, the period of transition from hospital discharge to life at home can represent a whole new phase in one's life. "The exhilaration felt upon resuming your life may be somewhat shattered by the overwhelming frustration encountered in realizing how unprepared you are for making the transition," says Tom Watson, sixty-five, who had a stroke two years ago.

When he left the rehabilitation center, Tom found that he was no longer a patient in the formal sense, but he was still very sick. Life in the real world is unlike life in the hospital, where responsibilities are kept away. "At home, life happens all around you," he says, "and insists you become an active participant in it. As willing as you may be to do that, in many ways it's just not possible for some time."

No two strokes are the same; and no two people who have a stroke have the same problems in walking, talking, listening, and processing information and in seeing, hearing, and perceiving.

"Coming home from the hospital after a stroke is a balancing act. Doing what you always did takes three times as long and has to be done differently," Watson says. "I have the best family support anyone could ask for from my wife and children. Even my grandchildren helped by reading their books to me. Together we watched "Sesame Street" and I relearned the alphabet. Big Bird has new meaning for me!"

Watson, a former county commissioner in California, is outgoing and doesn't hesitate to tell someone he has aphasia. "When I tell someone I have aphasia and need them to repeat what they're saying, they're willing to cooperate.

Otherwise, some people will treat you differently—
especially when they don't know what you need from
them. Once they know, most people come through. Of
course, I don't always use the word *aphasia*. Sometimes I
just explain that I have difficulty in understanding words,"
he says.

Regaining your strength and skills, reclaiming your
independence, beginning again to make life's important
decisions about what you will do and how you will live
may mean at first moving from a bed to a chair or a
wheelchair, dressing and bathing, walking or moving
around, talking and reading—in general, starting with
the simple things.

Living with a physical condition that limits one or more
life functions—either for a short time or always—affects
most things you do every day. Everything will now take
more energy, effort, time, planning, patience, and the co-
operation of your family, friends, and other helpers. It
won't be easy, but get ready to do it—because that's what
this book is all about.

EVERYDAY LIVING

"It's best to take it a day at a time when putting your life in
order. It's something you work toward for many months
or even years before it happens," says Watson. "Your main
goal is to allow your body, mind, and soul to heal and
strengthen as much as possible. You'll soon find the right
balance between too little activity or pushing yourself to
the point of overexertion."

At first, some days seem a week long. "Things you want
to accomplish—dressing, eating, bathing, talking, and
catching words and their meaning—take longer than any-

one can imagine." Two or three trips to therapy sessions crowd an already-busy day. Watson says he listens to his body to avoid overwhelming fatigue. "When I begin to get to that point, I stop what I'm doing, try to keep all activity to a minimum, or go to sleep until I have regained my strength."

"After a stroke, you are using more energy than ever before just to get around, to talk and to listen, so it's important to pace yourself throughout the day by balancing light and heavy tasks. Arrange to have times that are stimulating and others in between that are quiet—to sit down, nap, or simply relax," Watson says. He recommends noticing the times and activities during the day when you become especially fatigued. "Often a pattern emerges which indicates when you could regularly use someone's assistance, and it helps the family to be able to plan to be available or arrange for a paid helper on a scheduled basis. When you conserve your energy, you can actually do more." (For energy-saving suggestions, see page 128 in Chapter Four, "A Family Endeavor.")

Let's start with the most basic activities: getting in and out of bed, bathing, dressing, taking medications, preparing breakfast, lunch, or a snack, exercise, walking or moving around the house, and going outside.

It's best to get out of bed and dress every day. Complete bed rest actually deconditions the body. It lowers the capacity of the heart's pumping rate, reduces lung capacity, and alters blood pressure. It also increases one's susceptibility to pneumonia. Instead of remaining in bed, it's healthier to rest and take short naps in a comfortable chair with your legs elevated, or return to bed to rest only as needed, particularly after you eat, bathe, do your exercises, walk, and at other times when you're feeling tired. When you don't feel like sleeping but want to relax, use the time to make phone calls, listen to music, look at a magazine, read the newspaper, watch television, or listen to the radio.

After a good night's sleep, the morning hours are the ideal time to schedule the activities that require the most energy—whether for therapy at home or away, exercise, household chores, preparing a meal or snack, doctor's appointments, driving, and doing errands. To get started in the morning, you may want to do slow stretches, range-of-motion exercises, and other prescribed exercises in bed, to ease away some of the stiffness experienced after sleep. Some of these exercises are described later in this chapter on pages 70–74.

Before actually sitting up in bed, prepare first by rolling from side to side. This will involve both sides of the body. Before actually moving out of the bed, take your time, and plan ahead before going from one place to the next, whether it is transferring out of the bed into a wheelchair or standing up, getting in and out of the bathtub or into a car. By moving slowly and not making abrupt changes in your position, you are less likely to become dizzy. Many people find that taking two or three minutes to feel the ground under their feet before actually getting up is a good way to gain a greater sense of balance. If a spatial shoe, leg brace, sling, or splint is prescribed, you should put it on before standing. For more about transferring safely, see pages 66–70, later in this chapter.

If you feel rested and someone is available to assist you, the late morning may be a good time to take a sponge bath, a regular bath, or a shower. Because it is difficult to sit down and get up easily from the bathtub, most people prefer to sit on a bathtub transfer bench which has a back and adjustable legs. If you prefer to shower, you can purchase a bath chair that fits inside in an enclosed shower. Either way, you can be seated and have the advantage of getting out of the bathtub more easily on your own or when assisted. Remember to adjust the legs or seat to a height that is approximately the same as your wheelchair—if you use one—to ensure a safe transfer.

Always let your feet touch the floor of the bathtub or shower. If you feel unsteady in it, use a seat belt or any kind of belt that makes you feel more secure.

Try using a bath mitt and liquid soap rather than a washcloth, which must be held for use. Similarly, liquid soap from a dispenser hung on a wall shelf of the shower or tub is more manageable than a bar of soap. Long-handled sponges and brushes are also practical.

After getting out of the bathtub or shower, put on a terry-cloth robe and sit down to rest for a few moments. If you feel tired or agitated, lie down. Wait awhile before getting dressed, and continue only after you are relaxed. (More information about the proper methods for transferring in and out of the bathtub may be found later in this chapter on page 69.)

Have your clothes laid out the night before. To avoid fatigue, keep to a minimum reaching or bending for clothing in the closet. When your closets, dresser drawers, and cabinets are all arranged so you can easily reach clothing, towels, and other items, you will have a greater sense of independence.

Sit down on a steady chair or on the bed while you get dressed. Choose comfortable, easy-to-put-on clothes, such as jogging suits and sneakers with Velcro, which can be worn outdoors (for errands, visits to the doctor, and such) as well as inside.

Try to have the kitchen arranged so that you can easily reach dishes, pans, and any other items that you use often. You may want to use a stool with casters or a wheelchair to avoid standing while preparing meals. To save steps, use a rolling cart to take dishes to the sink or dishwasher or to bring food to the table. It's best to sit at a table or a counter when taking your meals rather than eating in bed. Whenever possible, make breakfast, lunch, or snacks for yourself.

When you have an appointment in the morning and

need to be out of the house at a certain time, attempt to do as much preparation as possible the night before. Set the table and ready the utensils, pans, and any food that doesn't need refrigeration. If you plan everything in advance and leave yourself enough time to rest after eating, you'll feel less rushed and more relaxed.

Your family may decide to create weekly menus for you or prepare dishes for the freezer that can be popped into a microwave or oven and be on the table in minutes. When there is good, appetizing food in the house, you'll feel less deprived by any new diet restrictions and it will be easier to stay on track.

Many people say that their favorite room is the bedroom and that they spend a great deal of time there relaxing, reading, and watching television. Try to create a bedroom or other room that meets your needs. It should be comfortable and quiet, and you should be able to get in and out of it easily, with closets arranged so that you can reach your clothes independently. Any furniture that interferes with your ability to get from place to place with ease should be rearranged. Chairs that are about nineteen or twenty inches high are easiest to get in and out of. If extra height is needed, place a pillow on chairs or a sofa, purchase leg extenders, or use wooden blocks available from a lumberyard.

If you live in a house with more than one floor, going up and down the stairs may be out of the question or may be very tiring, and your doctor may recommend that you limit the number of times you climb the stairs. Keep extra medications, an extra pair of eyeglasses, or any other items you need on both floors, so you or someone else doesn't have to keep on making trips in either direction to retrieve them. You may want to convert a living room or dining room on the first floor into a bedroom. (See Chapter Three, "Being Safe," for more detailed suggestions about making your home more accessible.)

ORIENT YOURSELF WITH TIME

Time plays a crucial role in our lives. Whether we're on the job or running a household, we are always conscious of our need to be on time and to make the most of the time we have. We use time to orient ourselves. For example, when we wake up in the middle of the night, the first thing we invariably think about is what time it is.

"Being aware of time is really important. This is especially true after a stroke: guide yourself by thinking of everything you do around time," says Vajaya Gadre, an occupational therapist. "Building a structure into your day, knowing what you're going to do until it becomes second nature, lets you be more accountable to yourself and others."

Ms. Gadre makes the following recommendations about time and how to manage it to best effect:

- **Awareness of time helps to organize the whole day**. If you or a family member records how much time it takes you to accomplish everyday activities, such as getting up, bathing, dressing, exercises, and eating, you can then estimate the time you need for your daily routine without ever feeling rushed. It's not a test of your abilities; it's simply a way of gathering information to add quality to your day.

- **Being aware of time will help you follow your schedule**. We think of everything we do in terms of time, whether it's morning, afternoon, or evening. We are accustomed to doing certain things at set times. Even when there is difficulty with the concept of time, if you connect the things you do with it, you will develop a structure to your day. Such structure has built-in discipline and accountability, so you are more likely to feel good about yourself when you *own* your own time.

- **Use calendars and daily reminders**. You may want to fill in a monthly calendar to remind you of coming events and appointments. A daily reminder is a good choice for tracking your daily activities and the medications you need to take at certain designated intervals. In addition, the family can create a message center in a handy location for notes and reminders. The most popular place is on a table or wall nearest to a phone, such as in the kitchen.
- **Digital watches and clocks are easier to read than their analog counterparts**. The whole time, such as "8:45 A.M.," can be seen at a glance, so you may find these easier to understand. Some people set an alarm as a reminder to take their medications and to keep track of other things they wish to remember.
- **It's easier to set realistic goals when you focus on time**. We are better able to harness our energies around goals when we are conscious of time. It helps us to prioritize activities and then apportion our time accordingly. When you have positive attitudes toward time, you will find it an ally, and not something you need to compete with.

Creating a Schedule That Suits You

Most people find it takes less energy and creates an opportunity to promote both self-sufficiency and healing to have a schedule that is maintained every day, perhaps with some variation on the weekend. For example, you may want to jot down those times when you have discomfort or pain and discuss this with your doctor and therapists. By keeping a schedule, it may be easier to discover which factors are triggering the pain. Perhaps a change in the dosage of your medicine is indicated. The doctor and therapists may be able to make recommendations or tell you what others have done to obtain relief.

On the next page is a sample of a chart that provides an informal schedule. You may want to keep a record of your blood pressure, blood sugar, medications, and any comments you would like to share with your doctor and therapists. You can create a chart that best suits your own needs, using the chart given as a guide.

BUILDING AND ENCOURAGING COMMUNICATION

"It's like waking up in Thailand," says Tom Watson, who has continued with speech therapy long after the formal sessions ended. He also attends an aphasia group once a week and uses computer software designed for people with aphasia, which helps him relearn basic language skills. He believes that recovery can be a lengthy, ongoing process. "Initially, you receive speech and language therapy, and this is an important first step to regaining skills and adapting to problems. But it doesn't stop there. You keep at it always, until you get back what you've lost."

Men and women who have had a stroke describe their anguish when trying to say "Please give me a glass of water" and having it come out "Put the store in the table" or "Wile dee dare ung pender glissen." They may find that they are unable to understand what is said or seen, or find that their ability to write, spell, gesture, or speak is impaired. Aphasia does not affect intelligence. People who have survived a stroke remain mentally alert, even though their speech may be—either temporarily or always—difficult to comprehend because it is jumbled, fragmented, slurred, or totally incoherent. "In thinking of these trying days," Tom Watson says, "you have to sit

Time	Informal Schedule	Blood Pressure	Pulse	Medicine	Comments
8:30 A.M.	Wake up; take a resting blood pressure, if possible. Medicine before and after breakfast; check off on medication chart				
9:00 A.M.	Breakfast; relax/read the newspaper/watch TV/make phone calls				
10:30 A.M.	Take a shower or a sponge bath; put on a terry robe, rest, then get dressed				
11:15 A.M.	Medicine, if any; check off on medication chart; rest/read the newspaper; make phone calls				
12:00 Noon	Walk or prepare lunch; relax; eat lunch; medicine, if any; check off on your chart				
2:00 P.M.	Relax; medicine; check off on chart; plan dinner				
4:00 P.M.	Take a walk; take pulse afterward; make a note of it				
4:30 P.M.	Watch television/read the newspaper; make phone calls/see friends; have a snack; medicine, if any; check it off on your chart; write down time/medication				
6:00 P.M.	Eat dinner				
7:00 P.M.	Relax				
8:30 P.M.	Get ready for bed; take medicines before bed; check it off on your chart; bedtime				

down with yourself, with your faith, and say, 'This too shall pass.' "

Almost all people with aphasia have some difficulty understanding spoken language. For example, some people may not associate the spoken word with an object or picture. "I may ask him to pass me his plate and get a fork," says the wife of a stroke survivor. She says this is where family members play a vital role in encouraging communication and reestablishing the self-esteem that is lost in this devastating experience.

Communication involves speaking as well as listening, understanding, reading, and writing. For someone who has had a left-hemisphere stroke, there may be difficulties in understanding conversation, speaking, gesturing, concentrating, listening, reading, or writing. The person also may have a right-sided weakness or paralysis.

For the person who has had a right-hemisphere stroke, there may be problems with using good judgment, concentration, memory, or reasoning. This person may speak excessively, be self-involved, find that time and space concepts are difficult, and neglect the left side of the body or environment.

Watson, who had a left-hemisphere stroke, has had difficulty speaking, reading, writing, and spelling. He feels his family has been especially helpful in dealing with his aphasia. "My wife and others in my family give me time to answer, without jumping in when it takes me some time to find the right words. I'm included in conversations, not made to feel I'm outside of what is being said. It's important to me that I can join in when and if I want. They ask me if I need help, and I feel comfortable asking them or anyone else to repeat something I don't understand. Family gatherings can get hectic, so it's understood that I might not stay around. I much prefer talking one-on-one."

Families who are making the adjustment to a loved one with aphasia are most successful when they encourage communication in some of the following ways:

- Family members and other caregivers should use simple sentences.
- A normal tone of voice is more effective than one that is excessively loud.
- Comprehension is best when there is no pause between words. On the other hand, when there is a pause between phrases or sentences, their meaning is more easily grasped.
- Questions should be phrased simply, so that they can be responded to with yes or no answers.
- Never force anyone to answer; rather, *encourage* a response.
- Because it takes a great deal of energy for someone who has aphasia to talk and process information, it's best to engage in conversations when they are receptive—preferably, when they're rested and relaxed.
- Since communication is the goal, it is inappropriate to correct grammar or pronunciation. More about materials to encourage communication and reintroduce the return of language is on page 236.

PROPER POSITIONING

At all times—whether lying in bed, sitting, or walking—proper body positioning is essential for maintaining the body's "integrity," that is, the basic wholeness and soundness of the body. Proper positioning of the body will help to prevent the development of contractures, which are a shortening of muscles around the joints. While in the hospital, the nursing staff and the physical and occupational therapists teach proper positioning to a person who has had a stroke; they also advise family members and other helpers. Here are some reminders for proper positioning. Your physical therapist may have instructions and illustrations that would be helpful for you and your family in maintaining correct posture.

- **The head and neck need to be in alignment to maintain balance.** The position of your head affects the muscle tone of your trunk, arms, and legs. If the position of your head is turned to one side, it may impede your balance and your ability to move about. You might find it helpful to use a mirror to see how to center your head with your shoulders.
- **Position yourself so your weight is evenly distributed.** When sitting, bend at the hips, not the lower back. Distribute your weight on both sides, rather than placing weight on only one hip. If you find you have a tendency to lean more to one side, prop up that side with pillows or a foam wedge. While lying on the affected side, lean slightly backward with the pillows behind your back, so that your affected arm is extended. Lean slightly forward when lying on the sound side and stretch the affected arm forward on a pillow placed under your arm to prevent the shoulder from hyperextending.
- **Your affected shoulder can easily become painfully dislocated without proper support.** To hold your shoulder joint in place, support your forearm with a pillow. Slide the shoulder blade away from the spine, allowing the shoulder and arm to stretch forward. Lift the weaker wrist with the sound hand to pull the arm forward. If you have swelling in the upper arm, elevate the entire arm, and support it all the way up to the armpit with pillows.
- **Keep the elbow straight, and position the palm up.** The elbow should be kept straight, or slightly bent, whenever possible. The forearm and hand

are positioned with the palm up, even when the arm must be close to the chest and the hand is on the lap.

- **The wrist should be extended backward, keeping your fingers as straight as possible.** Sometimes an occupational therapist recommends a splint to support the fingers. Ask the therapist for exercises to reduce tightness, or perhaps a device to reduce excessive muscle tone. Avoid placing a ball in the palm to increase strength, unless this has been recommended, to avoid the possible development of contractures at the fingers.

- **Hips, knees, and ankles should not roll outward when sitting.** Choose a chair low enough so your feet can be flat on the floor and allows you to sit at the right angle. If you use a wheelchair, and one leg helps to move the chair, place your other foot on the footrest to help support it. When sitting in the wheelchair, make sure that your hips and knees are flexed at about 90 degrees by adjusting the footrests.

- **Family members can help you to keep proper posture.** Change your position often. Lift your leg to reposition your foot when it drops down, and raise your affected arm with your sound arm to realign your position. When you are changing position, bring your affected arm in toward your body as you're moving. Family members and other helpers can assist you in checking your body alignment.

- **When you walk, practice exercises to correct muscle imbalance.** If you have voluntary movement in your arm, it should hang free during walking. If your shoulder is mildly dislocated, a sling may be recommended for walking. If your affected leg tends to turn outward, instead of your foot and knee facing forward when you walk, your physical therapist may give you exercises to correct the muscle imbalance.

- **Protect your skin by changing positions frequently.** To avoid pressure sores and breakdown of skin, shift your position frequently to increase blood flow and to regain correct balance. Bedding and undergarments must be kept dry to protect the skin. Choose a soothing lotion for a therapeutic massage to increase circulation.
- **Bridging provides a way to change positions on your own.** Bridging gets its name because you literally make a bridge with your body by lifting the buttocks off the bed. Careful instruction is needed from the physical therapist to perform the bridging exercise correctly. It is important to correctly position the arms so that your shoulders are supported. Both legs are bent with the knees together, while your feet are planted firmly on the bed to carry some of the weight. At first, you may need help to place and hold the affected foot and knee in the required position and to lift your hips.

The affected shoulder needs to be well positioned and comfortable. Only the lower arm is rolled inward. As you lift your hips, the increased pressure on your forearms and hands begin important weight-bearing benefits and—at the same time—the shoulders roll outward.

As you lift your hips off the bed, you bring the trunk muscles on the affected side into action, thus starting active exercise in hip control. These primary trunk movements are the first to return. From there, recovery spreads downward—from trunk to the hip, knee, and foot; and from the trunk to the shoulder, elbow, wrist, and hand. This establishes strong and controlled hip movement, which in turn affects standing up, sitting down, and walking, as well as promoting greater self-sufficiency.

The exercise helps to prevent the buildup of unwanted reflex activity, known as spasticity. Once this

exercise can be done on one's own, whenever a read-
justment of position is desired, it can be done independently.

Preparing to Transfer (Moving Safely from One Place to Another)

- **Before beginning the transfer, plan ahead.** Take
  your time. Visualize how you will go from one place
  to a wheelchair or standing up; then slowly get up
  and make your transfer.
- **Everything that could cause an accident must be
  moved out of the way.** Furniture, rugs, or anything
  underfoot should be moved out of the way.
- **When transferring from the bed to a wheelchair,
  both should be kept stationary.** If the bed is on
  casters, have it pushed against the wall. The brakes of
  the wheelchair must be locked on each side.
- **Both you and your helper need to signal each
  other.** It is a good idea for you and your helper to tell
  each other what you are going to do during the transfer. Your helper should never rush you and should
  allow you enough time to accomplish each step in a
  careful, methodical manner.
- **Feel the ground under your feet before getting
  up.** Before moving, sit at the edge of the bed for two
  or three minutes with your feet on the floor, and
  make sure you feel strong enough to balance without
  becoming dizzy. By moving slowly and not making
  abrupt changes in your position, you are less likely to
  become light-headed. Your toes need to be pointing
  straight ahead for the best balance—not outward or
  inward.

- **Have a cane within reach on your sound side.** If you use a cane, have it at the ready. Your weight should be equally balanced on both legs with the cane giving support.
- **Do as much of the work as you can when transferring.** The helper is there to keep your body in proper alignment and to give you a feeling of security. If necessary, you can be lifted by one or more helpers, but it is the least-safe method of transfer and the one that affords the least self-sufficiency.

  Your helper supports your back, shoulders, and under your elbows to keep the arm in the shoulder socket as you move from one place to the next. If a shoulder sling has been prescribed, put it on before you attempt to stand up. A good way to support your affected arm is for helpers to place one hand behind the shoulder, the other holding your hand in a handshake grasp. Your elbow is bent, and the helper is in a forward position, being careful not to pull you backward.
- **Helpers must guard against hurting their own backs or losing their balance.** To lessen the strain and prevent back injury, the helper should keep hips and knees slightly bent when helping you into a standing position. It is less of a strain on the back muscles if helpers use their leg muscles—which are meant to carry the weight of lifting. For extra security, a safety belt can be used, especially outdoors where the terrain is often uneven and bumpy.

  Planting their feet firmly on the ground, helpers bend their knees, using their knees to brace your knees, while their shoulders keep your shoulders in place, as you move from one place to the next.
- **To ensure safety and efficiency, it is best to have the assistant be in the right position.** This is accomplished by the assistant standing close to you. If you

and your helper stand apart, strain is placed on the
helper's back. The assistant stands with a broad base
of support by keeping his or her feet slightly apart,
with one foot ahead of the other. This position allows
the assistant to maintain balance and quickly and
easily to shift his or her weight whenever necessary.

- **Move toward your stronger side during the transfer.** The helper approaches you from your sound
  side. From the front, the helper supports your
  weaker shoulder and moves it forward, while you put
  weight on your sound arm in preparation for sitting
  up. If the wheelchair faces the foot of the bed when
  you transfer out of the bed, then the wheelchair will
  face the head of the bed when you want to return to
  bed.
- **You need to see the place toward which you're
  moving.** The helper needs to take care not to block
  your view so that you can see where you need to
  move to.
- **A two-foot-long sliding board can be used to negotiate difficult transfers.** If you are unable to
  stand or would feel safer negotiating transfers of two
  different heights or involving some distance—such
  as from the wheelchair to a car—a sliding board can
  be very helpful.
- **Make sure the footrest is off when you transfer, if
  you propel the wheelchair.** The other footrest
  should be left on to support your leg. When a cane is
  used, have it stand on the foot plate.
- **There is a tendency to lean backward when
  changing positions.** To move into the correct position and to make it easier for someone to assist you,
  lean slightly forward when transferring.
- **Helpers may be fearful of harming the people
  they assist.** While helpers must be careful not to pull
  or twist your arms or legs or place you in an uncomfortable position, it is equally important that helpers

support and touch your affected arm and leg. Then they can become more aware of that side of your body and involve it in all activities.

Physical therapists, occupational therapists, and visiting nurses can show you and your helper the proper body mechanics for transferring and using the wheelchair.

ASSISTANCE IN THE BATHROOM

Performing an Assisted Wheelchair Transfer to the Toilet

When helping in a transfer from a wheelchair to the toilet, the assistant should bring the wheelchair as close to the front edge of the toilet as possible. The brakes of the wheelchair should be locked and the footrests swung to the outside.

The body weight of the person being assisted is borne entirely or as much as possible on the stronger leg, and the trunk is bent slightly downward to establish a center of gravity closer to the grab bar on the wall.

The stronger side should be brought nearest to the toilet. The person being assisted can grab hold of the handrail firmly with the stronger arm, using it to pull up to a standing position, with or without some help.

Performing an Assisted Transfer to the Bathtub

It takes good balance and sure footing to get in and out of the bathtub. And it is generally more difficult to get *out* of the tub on your own than to get into it. The transfer is made toward the weaker side, so that when you return from the tub, you can move with your stronger side first. If it is too difficult, a sliding board may help to lessen the risk of falling.

A sturdy chair (if possible, the same height as the bath chair) should be placed outside of the tub. Use the bars on the walls for greater security when lifting yourself to a sitting position on the chair in the tub, or have assistance ready in helping to place you on the bath chair.

If you use a wheelchair, have the brakes locked and place it as close as possible to the bath chair, while the assistant firmly holds the chair.

RANGE-OF-MOTION EXERCISES

Range-of-motion exercises can keep joints moving freely and fully. You probably remember that you started almost immediately to do these or similar exercises to prevent deformities and loss of full motion of a joint.

What follows in this section are some of the range-of-motion exercises that you can do either by yourself or with someone assisting you. Your physical therapist should be able to give you written instructions and demonstrate to you and someone assisting you how to do these and other prescribed exercises. Be sure that you know how often the exercises should be done and at what intervals—and follow this schedule as carefully as you can.

Some families find it helpful to bring a video camera to therapy sessions to have a record that they can follow at home. If you think this would be helpful, discuss with your physical therapist the possibility of choosing a convenient time to record your progress.

Points for Assistants in Range-of-Motion Exercises

Do all exercises in a slow, smooth motion. Create a relaxed, unhurried, and calm atmosphere. It is a time of partnership between you and the person you are assisting. The exercises work best if you encourage feedback by communicating freely.

The assistant firmly holds the joint being exercised with one hand and uses the other hand to create and guide the movement that is desired. The person who is assisting stops the exercise when he or she feels that the joint is no longer moving freely, or when the person being assisted feels pressure or discomfort.

Shoulder-and-Arm Exercise (over the Head)

The assistant stands at your side, by your shoulder, and your arm is straight at your side with your thumb up. The assistant places one hand on your elbow to support it and uses the other hand to hold your hand. The assistant lifts your arm over your head, toward your ear, keeping your elbow straight, then returns your arm to the starting position.

Shoulder-and-Arm Exercise (to the Side)

The starting position begins with the assistant standing by your shoulder. The assistant places one hand above your elbow and holds your hand with his or her other hand. The assistant then moves your arm away from your side, around toward your ear—keeping your elbow straight, with your palm up, and your arm parallel to the floor. The assistant then returns your arm to the starting position.

Shoulder-and-Elbow Exercise

Standing by your elbow, the assistant places your arm at your side, with the elbow bent so your fingers are pointing toward the ceiling.

The assistant then places one hand above your elbow and holds your hand with his or her other hand. Then they lift your upper arm so that your hand moves across your chest. The assistant then turns your upper arm outward so that your hand moves away from your chest, then returns your arm to the starting position.

Elbow-Bending Exercise

The assistant stands at your elbow and places your arm straight at your side, with your thumb up. The assistant places one hand above your elbow and holds your hand, bending your elbow so that your hand goes toward your shoulder. The assistant then returns your arm to the starting position.

Note: The physical therapist may recommend that you do additional elbow forearm-turning, wrist-bending, and other exercises and can give you instructions as well as demonstrate them.

Finger-Bending and Straightening Exercise

The assistant stands by your elbow and places your arm at your side with the elbow bent and the fingers pointing toward the ceiling.

Placing one hand palm down over the back of your hand, the assistant uses the other hand to support your wrist, and helps you make a tight fist. The assistant then assists you in straightening your fingers so that your hand is flat, returning your hand to the starting position.

Hip and Knee-Bending Exercise

The assistant stands by your knee. Placing your leg out straight on the bed, with the kneecap pointing toward the ceiling, the assistant places one hand under your knee and the other hand under your heel. The assistant bends your knee toward your chest, then returns your leg to the starting position.

Leg Exercise (to the Side)

Standing by your knee, the assistant places your leg out straight on the bed, with the kneecap pointing toward the ceiling. The assistant places one hand under your knee and the other hand under your heel, moving your leg away from the other leg. The knee is kept straight and the toes are pointing upward. In order to move your leg all the way out to the side, the assistant may have to take a step backward. The assistant then returns your leg to the starting position.

Leg-Raising Exercise

Standing by your knee, the assistant places your leg out straight on the bed, with the kneecap pointing toward the ceiling. Placing one hand under your knee and one hand under your heel, the assistant lifts your leg up toward your chest, while keeping the knee straight. The assistant then returns your leg to the starting position.

Foot Exercise

The assistant stands by your foot and places your leg out straight on the bed, with the toes pointing upward. Your heel is cupped in the palm of the assistant's hand, with the ball of your foot resting against the assistant's arm. The assistant's other hand is on top of your ankle.

Your foot is brought up by the assistant pulling down on your heel and using an arm to press on the ball of your foot. As the assistant's arm relaxes, your foot returns to the starting position. You can point your foot down by pressing up on your heel and down on your foot. Your foot is then brought back to the starting position, with your toes pointing toward the ceiling. For a video to follow when exercising, send for *Stroke Survivor's Workout* from the American Heart Stroke Connection (800) 553-6321.

SKIN CARE

A person who has had a stroke, and a care-giving family member or other helper, must be vigilant about inspecting the skin for redness, swelling, and signs of inflammation. Injury to the skin can take place by bumping an arm or leg that lacks sensation or by crushing fingers in the spokes of the wheelchair, particularly when transferring. When changing position or in a transfer, the helper must *lift* the person across the sheet. Pulling the person can cause friction injuries and pressure sores. When using a wheelchair, change position by pushing up while supporting your weight on an armrest. Smooth out the clothing under you and immediately change any clothing that is wet or damp from incontinence or perspiration.

   Pressure sores and skin breakdown can occur when
there is a lack of frequent turning or changing positions in
bed. When you remain in bed for any extended period of
time—especially when poor circulation, decreased sensation, diabetes, or fragile skin are involved—turning or
repositioning the body should take place **at least** every
two hours. By taking a few extra moments to examine the
area on which you have been lying for redness and integrity of the skin, you may prevent the possibility of skin
breakdown later on. Keeping the skin clean and dry and
massaging the skin and bony prominences with lotion are
beneficial measures in maintaining the skin's integrity.
   When you do notice skin breakdown from a pressure
sore or bruise, immediate medical attention is necessary.
Your doctor or a visiting nurse can recommend ways to
alleviate the problem and prescribe medication and treatment.

STAN SHAPIRO, ACCOUNTANT

Since my stroke, it takes three or four times the effort to do things, even simple things that a two-year-old kid can do. You just have to see the humor in it and push on. You know, like when I wash dishes. Initially, when I had a fork or another utensil in my hand, I'd wash the front of it, but I couldn't flip it over to the back. So I'd have to put down the sponge and turn it over in my hand. And this is what made everything double the time.

> "You have to think, 'I'm going to get better and I'm going to make the best of what I have . . .' "

You think sometimes, "Why can't things come easily to me?" But you have to understand what you went through was really quite something. You had a lot taken away from you, but you're building yourself back up again with the help of some positive thinking. I'm going to do it. There's no problem here; I'm going to do it. When the doctors say there's plenty of room for improvement, I feel good. I'm trying to help myself. God helps those who help themselves. You can't give up with anything. What worked for me, in large part, was thinking positively. You have to think, I'm going to get better and I'm going to make the best of what I have, at the present time.

What used to be important to me was the well-being of the family. And I guess I kind of pushed my own health aside. It was never uppermost, and took a backseat to security. You know, you work, you put in extra hours, overtime—even when you didn't get paid, because you're thinking this would help you solidify your position, guarantee your security. At this point, well, I realize that without my health, there is no security. Now I have to consider my health first in anything that I do.

Thinking about myself first is one of the toughest things for me to do, because I'm always accustomed to doing for other people. For example, for year after year—don't ask me why—I never put a cover on our swimming pool, so every year I'd have to clean it out. And most of the time I'd be doing it by myself. Now, I can't do it. So my kids finally caught the drift of what's going on, and they decided well, if we're going to have a swimming pool this year, we better get our friends down to help clean it out. So today they cleaned it out, and we're filling it now. The fact is now because of the way I'm thinking—I force myself to think of *me* first. I don't feel bad about it; I thought I would, but I don't. In fact, I feel pretty good that other people are chipping in.

After my stroke, I returned to my bowling league. I attempted to restore my normal routine as much as possible, even though now I only keep score there. Anyway, when I was first walking down the steps to the alleys, somebody must have said, "Stan's coming." And suddenly the whole place breaks out singing the "Presidential March," with cheers and things like that. It was very touching, and in fact, I started to cry a little bit.

Chapter Three

Being Safe

It's not whether you get knocked down. It's whether you get up again.

—VINCE LOMBARDI

Home Safe Home

While a family member is in the hospital, many families start thinking about making changes in the house or apartment that will provide added comfort, accessibility, and safety for their loved one. A few families, especially homeowners with a family member who uses a wheelchair, may decide to make extensive changes.

For example, if the house is on two floors and there is an inaccessible bedroom on the second floor, the family may decide to transform the dining room or living room into a bedroom; install a ramp, elevator, or chairlift; or make a ground-level addition to the house itself. Some families decide not to remain in their present home for any number of reasons. It may be too costly or inaccessible, or the nearby transportation is insufficient or inconvenient for themselves or for paid helpers.

When a loved one lives alone in a two-story house, the family may decide to turn the second floor into an apartment to bring in additional income or to find a companion or helper who will share the space. A family may need to look for alternatives to a nursing home and consider the possibility of the person who had the stroke remaining at home with a personal-care attendant or moving in with a daughter, son, or other relative.

Home Accident Factors

Several factors that contribute to home accidents after hospitalization include:

- the aftereffects of surgery and illness
- medications that alter vision, perception, and cognition

- sensory distortions that can affect balance, judgment, recognition, and comprehension
- fatigue

Falls rank as the number-one cause of accidental home fatalities, particularly for people over sixty-five. Home accidents account for more injuries than motor-vehicle and workplace accidents *combined*. The National Safety Council estimates that close to four million disabling injuries each year are due to home accidents.

Two-thirds of all falls in the home occur at the floor level and are the result of someone tripping over an object or slipping on a wet surface—particularly on a tile floor after bathing. This is a particular concern for someone who has had a stroke. The Rusk Institute recommends that a family member make a room-by-room check to eliminate potential accident sites and create a safer, easier-to-navigate environment for the family member who has had a stroke.

Getting into Your Home

The following guidelines can help you prepare for the homecoming of someone who has had a stroke. Make sure that:

Walkways leading to the house are smooth.

- Check for deep cracks and broken areas in pavements and pathways; have them repaired to prevent accidents.
- Install gently sloping curb cuts.

The entrance is accessible.

- Ideally, the approach to the house should be fairly level, with only one or two steps.
- If a ramp is needed, it should be built on a ratio of 12 inches of length for each 1 inch of height and should

be at least 3 feet wide. Most people with two functioning upper arms can self-wheel at this ratio.
Someone pushing a wheelchair may be able to manage a slightly steeper incline.

- If doorbells, mailboxes, and peepholes are higher
than can be easily reached from chair height, adjust
them for a wheelchair user.
- A flashing light can be attached to the doorbell to
alert someone with a hearing disability to the presence of a person at the door.

Doors, Thresholds, and Hallways

Doors need to be wide enough to accommodate a wheelchair.

- Door openings should be at least 32 inches clear or
more to provide enough room for a person in a wheelchair to clear the entrance without harm to the arms.
- If the width is 29 inches, arms must be kept inside the
chair while someone assists in pushing the chair
through.
- A device is available for some nonmotorized wheelchairs to reduce the width of wheelchairs to allow
enough clearance for narrow doors.
- For added space, remove the molding or change the
hinges. If the doors are not wide enough, the molding
should be removed and the hinges changed so that
the door can be opened fully without interfering with
the entranceway.

Thresholds won't cause accidents.

- Thresholds higher than one-half-inch are barriers for
wheelchair users and someone using a cane. Most
thresholds can be entirely removed or beveled. A
wedge-shaped piece of wood can be attached to the

threshold, nailed down securely, and then covered
with a rubber mat to make the threshold easier to
cross.

Hallways need to be wide enough to maneuver a wheelchair in.

• Hallways should be at least 42 inches, but preferably
48 to 60 inches wide, so that wheelchair users will
have enough clearance to get into each room.

Steps and Elevators

Steps should be easy to climb and descend.

• Steps must afford secure footing. If carpeting covers
the steps, it must be securely fastened, with the first
and last step marked with a different color. Many
accidents occur because of uncertainty about the top
and bottom steps.
• Stairways should be well lighted, especially if a family member has impaired vision.
• Stair lifts or an elevator can make upper floors more
easily accessible. Stair lifts can be purchased or
rented, and some will accommodate a wheelchair.
For wheelchair clearance, allow for a space that is
more than 5 feet deep and 5 feet 6 inches wide. The
door needs a sensing device to prevent closure while
entering or exiting, with controls no more than 4 feet
from the elevator floor.

Handrails need to be installed on both sides of the stairs.

• Handrails should afford a firm grasp, be securely
anchored into the wall, and capable of withstanding
weight.

Thermostats, Electrical Switches, and Outlets

- Place thermostats and intercoms a maximum of 54 inches above the floor so that they can be easily reached by wheelchair users. Electrical outlets should be no less than 18 inches from the floor.
- Check lamps and electrical appliances for worn wiring and electrical outlets for overloading.
- Secure any telephone and other electrical cords; if possible, run them under a carpet.
- Three-pronged, grounded plugs are needed for medical equipment. Have an electrician check to see both if the electrical outlets in your home are equipped to receive grounded plugs and if the wiring is suitable for the equipment.
- If a motorized chair or a respirator is used, extra batteries should be on hand in the event of a power failure. Make sure that the replacement batteries are filled and charged. Many utility companies maintain lists of the names, addresses, and apartment numbers of people who may need assistance in the event of a power failure. You may call the utility company to ask them to charge batteries or to obtain electrical power for other equipment you are unable to use when you are without electricity.

The Bathroom

Have the vanity removed for open space below the sink.

- If you prefer to sit while grooming, the vanity should be taken out from under the sink or a portion cut out and the doors removed, to allow space for your legs when seated at the sink. Wrap the pipes under the sink to prevent your legs from being scraped or getting burned.

- Place toiletries in cabinets or baskets on either side of the sink to be within easy reach.
- If the mirror above the sink is too high, a wall extension mirror can be used.
- At least one bathroom in the house should have a 32-inch clearance space for the door opening and 5 feet by 5 feet of clear floor space for maneuvering a wheelchair around the bathroom.

Fixture and appliance controls should be easy to use and easily reached.

- Single levers on faucets require less wrist and finger motion than round knobs.
- Electrical switches, toilet-tissue dispensers, and towel racks should be placed at such a height that you do not lose your balance when reaching for them.
- If a wheelchair is used, chair height is measured by how far up something is before it can be reached. From a frontal approach, it is approximately 48 inches; a parallel approach is about 54 inches.
- Before installing anything permanently, try it out to make sure it's conveniently located for easy accessibility.
- A raised toilet seat may give greater independence since it can be purchased or constructed to make it easier to sit and stand up. However, a wheelchair user may prefer instead to have the toilet itself raised.
- A safety bar on the wall and on one or both sides of the toilet is useful and ensures safe transfers.
- If it is difficult to walk to the bathroom, arrange to have the bed in the vicinity of the bathroom or use a commode chair.

Use a bathtub transfer bench or shower chair.

- If sitting down and getting up while in the bathtub is difficult, try a bath chair with adjustable legs that you can sit on. If you prefer to shower, you can obtain a chair that fits inside an enclosed shower. Either way, you can be seated and have the advantage of getting out of the bathtub on your own, or more easily when assisted. Make sure the legs are adjusted to a comfortable height so your feet touch the floor of the bathtub or shower. If you feel unsteady in the chair, use a seat belt or any kind of belt that will make you feel more secure. Comparison shopping always saves money because of the wide price range to be found on similar items. (See pages 233–236 for a list of places where these and other useful personal and household items can be purchased.)

A hand-held showerhead is useful.

- A hand-held showerhead allows you or someone assisting you to safely test in advance the water temperature, as well as to regulate the water pressure for a pleasurable massage action. A hand-held showerhead also allows you to shampoo your hair and rinse it without the need to raise your hands above your head. This item can cost as little as $25 or more than $200, depending on the features. The more expensive models have a button to control water pressure in order to produce a soothing massage effect.
- Choose warm water over hot, so that you do not become dizzy or faint.
- Use a long-handled bath sponge or brush to reach your back and feet without bending.

Install a reinforced safety bar.

- Safety bars definitely should be installed at the appropriate height for getting in and out of the tub or shower. The bolts must be reinforced into the wall studs rather than only the tile surface, so that they support your weight without coming loose. Some safety bars clamp directly onto the tub; these can be found in housewares and home-care supply stores, as well as in a number of mail-order catalogs.

Apply nonskid strips in the tub and use rubber mats.

- Most accidents in the bathroom take place when someone slips in or around the tub or on a wet tile floor. Towels or thin mats wrinkle and can cause you to lose your footing, particularly when moving about is difficult. Try covering the tile floor with rubber-backed carpeting, making sure that it lies flat. Place a rubber mat or rubber-backed bath mat on the floor adjacent to the tub.

Have extra hooks installed near the tub.

- Clothing, towels, or a robe can be kept in the bathroom on hooks hung low enough so that you can reach them easily.

Consider using an over-the-head terry-cloth poncho or robe instead of toweling dry.

- You expend less energy putting it on, and it keeps you comfortable and presentable if you decide not to dress right away.

An intercom provides needed assistance when no one is available to stay nearby while you are in the bathroom.

• You may want to have someone stay with you in the bathroom or close by when you bathe. Or you can install an inexpensive intercom which can be purchased at stores such as Radio Shack. That way, if you are in the bathroom on your own and need or want something, the intercom is right there. Intercoms are often set up in the bedroom, bathroom, and kitchen. Each house has its own requirements, particularly if there is more than one floor.

Keep a night-light in and near the bathroom.

• Have a night-light on during the night in the hall leading to the bathroom and in other rooms that you are likely to use at night. Inexpensive night-lights are available that are automatically activated when you turn the lights off.

Medications must be clearly marked, especially when several are prescribed.

• To avoid confusion, medications need to be identified. (For more about medications, see page 156 in Chapter Five, "Taking Charge of Your Health.") Substances such as bleach and cleaning fluid, which would be harmful if mistakenly ingested, must be clearly labeled and kept safely away from medications, particularly if a family member is visually impaired or disoriented.

• Some medications or a combination of medications may alter and distort touch, taste, and perception or increase vision, hearing, and sensory deficits; they

also may compromise balance, judgment, recognition, and comprehension.

The Bedroom

Raise your own bed to a comfortable height.

- If you prefer to use your own bed but you and the
  people assisting find it is too low, get a few wooden
  blocks from a lumberyard to raise the bed to the
  height you prefer. A comfortable height is usually 18
  to 22 inches from the floor to the top of the mattress.
- Try your bed at different heights to see which one is
  easiest and safest for transferring. With a bed that is
  high, it is easier to sit down and stand up from the
  edge without help. A bed that is too low places a
  strain on the back of the helper when changing your
  position or lifting during transfers.
- If the mattress is too soft to give leverage to lift yourself more easily to a sitting position, plywood placed
  between the mattress and box spring provides extra
  firmness.
- Wheels under the box spring should be locked and
  stabilized against the wall.
- If a hospital bed is used, the brakes can be locked for
  additional security.
- A wedge pillow can support your back when you are
  sitting up. Extra pillows will help support an arm or
  shoulder and maintain proper body alignment. (For
  more about positioning, see page 62 in Chapter Two,
  "Recovering at Home.")

You may consider renting a motorized bed.

- In the early months of recovery, a single motorized
  bed you can raise and lower—similar to those used
  in hospitals—may be more comfortable than a

double bed and can make it easier for family members to assist you in changing your position and getting in and out of bed. Home-care supply companies and pharmacies usually rent beds on a monthly basis. Check your local Yellow Pages for a listing of suppliers. Do some comparison shopping before renting, since you may find rental charges for a motorized bed run anywhere from $100 to more than $250 a month, for virtually the same type of bed.

Use adjustable closet shelves.

• Gain greater self-sufficiency by arranging the closet so that you can easily reach your clothing. A wire shelving package, which usually includes closet rods, can be installed and adjusted to any height. Add-on baskets can be attached to replace cabinets and increase storage space without cluttering a room. Hand-manipulated "reachers" can aid in getting down clothes stored on high shelves.

Modify or replace hardware so that it is easier to use.

• Levers are easier to manage than round fixtures and knobs. For dresser drawers that are difficult to open and close, try looping a cord around the knobs for easy pulling.

Avoid accidents by eliminating obstacles.

• Clothing, furniture, and other obstacles may need to be rearranged to avoid tripping over them. (For more about potential accident sites and personal safety, see page 82.)

The Kitchen

Arrange the kitchen for maximum efficiency.

- Try to arrange the kitchen so that dishes, pans, and food in the refrigerator or freezer can be easily reached.
- To avoid bending or standing while preparing meals, use a wheelchair or a chair with casters. Cabinets can be lowered, and sliding or bifold doors that take up less room are a good choice for cabinets and cupboards.
- A rolling cart saves steps when taking dishes to the sink or dishwasher or when bringing food to the table.
- There are many advantages to getting out of bed as soon as possible, because movement and activity are beneficial and promote the healing process. For example, it's best to sit at a table or a counter when eating meals, instead of staying in bed. You will find getting up can give you an emotional boost as well.

Allow adequate space to move around in.

- Ideally, the kitchen is U- or L-shaped or has an open floor plan with sufficient space in which to maneuver a wheelchair. The heights of the counter, sink, and stove should be between 30 to 40 inches.
- Consider removing some of the lower cabinets to provide more room both for turning and for knee spaces under the sink or countertops.
- If wall cabinets are too high, lower them and add some new cabinets or a free standing storage cabinet.
- If countertops are high, use instead a cart with wheels for food preparation. It can be rolled to the stove and refrigerator and can also double as a serving cart.

- A drawer set with a plank of wood across it can provide a low work surface for use as a cutting board or bowl holder.
- Use a microwave oven. If a countertop range is used, be careful not to burn yourself when reaching over the burners.
- If you are seated while preparing food, the stove, sink, and counters need to be at a height to allow everything to be within easy reach.
- To provide space for your legs under the sink while seated, have the cabinet removed and wrap exposed pipes.

Use adaptive devices to make work easier.

- When working in the kitchen, a cutting board designed for one-handed use will hold bread and other food in place for cutting.
- Special kinds of knives are available to make cutting possible when using one hand. Forks, spoons, and cooking utensils that are easy to grasp and provide self-sufficiency also can be purchased. (For sources, see Chapter Seven, "Information, Services, and Products," page 234.)

WHAT FAMILIES NEED TO KNOW

Arthur Marantz was eager to resume his life after three weeks in the hospital, but he and his wife, Bryna, were apprehensive. He was transferred from the hospital to a community rehabilitation institute for one month, then continued his treatment three times a week with a physical therapist, occupational therapist, and speech therapist. "From the physical therapist we know the work-out to do, from the speech therapist we know what speech exercises to do, and the doctor wrote prescriptions for the medications and assistive devices," says Bryna. "But when at last we were home on our own, we felt very uncertain about how we were going to handle by our-selves the services that an entire staff of professionals had once provided."

In the early months of Arthur's recovery at home, Bryna felt always on the alert, and her husband called her "the bodyguard." Several times he fell. Not only did he fall several times, but he also constantly bumped into things around the house and often hurt himself badly. She had heard of a few people who broke their hips after a stroke, so she sharpened her vigil. This concern even interrupted her sleep. She would be awakened when Arthur got up to go to the bathroom or wanted to change his position in bed, which he couldn't do without her help. It reminded her of a time when their children were very young and she developed the habit of "sleeping with the third ear."

Bryna's main concern centered on how she would know when a change in her husband's condition indicated an emergency and what she would do. A visiting nurse alerted her to signs and symptoms of problems. Together they created an emergency plan and carefully wrote it out for her use, as well as for her husband and the personal-care attendant. Emergency numbers were posted in large block letters by the telephone.

Bryna's confidence increased as she learned more about stroke and aphasia from both the speech therapists and from pamphlets and books. Even before she and Arthur joined a stroke club, they started getting copies of the club's newsletter. Reading aloud the personal stories in the newsletter became an inspiration for them.

When a member of the family has a stroke, it means that everyone in the family must learn more about the

medical aspects of stroke so they can better judge when to
call the doctor. Understanding the condition helps families know they are capable of doing something to make a
difference.

In the event of an emergency, it is essential to obtain
immediate medical care for your loved one. Family members may rationalize that because their husband, wife, or
parent has a good doctor, they needn't concern themselves
about what to do if an emergency occurs. But you may be
the only person present at the time of an emergency and,
therefore, you must know what to do *before* the emergency medical service arrives.

In fact, a loved one may have a stroke, or a recurrence,
but because they are not experiencing any pain or any
other dramatic symptom, it may not appear to be a situation in which time is crucial. Medical intervention at the
very onset can reduce the possible negative physical consequences.

Doctors believe it is essential for families to be able to
recognize the warning signs of an initial stroke or recurrence, to know what to do and not to do in an emergency,
to have a list ready of all prescribed medications, and be
able to supply emergency personnel with specific information about the condition or combination of conditions.
*Never delay getting help just to see if the stroke symptoms
abate by themselves, even if the stricken family member
resists calling for assistance.*

It's a good idea for family members to talk with the
primary-care physician or neurologist about both the specific symptoms and emergency signs of stroke and the
possible reactions from prescribed medications that need
to be reported. If there has been surgery, you and your
family must also know about the particular signs and
symptoms that should be reported to your doctor immediately. This information should be noted down for safe-
keeping and future reference.

THE WARNING SIGNS OF A STROKE

Because brain cells can die very quickly after a stroke, it is crucial to recognize warning signs of an impending stroke and to get to a hospital quickly for emergency medical intervention. Even seconds count when you consider that there are now, for example, new clot-dissolving drugs that can have a major impact on survival if administered promptly.

Since the brain controls hundreds of activities, the range of stroke symptoms is broad. Some warning signs of stroke are common and relatively easy to spot. Other signs are harder to detect, particularly a transient ischemic attack—also known as a "ministroke."

The rehabilitation staff at the Rusk Institute offers the following guidelines to families. During a stroke, most people have one or more of these symptoms:

- sudden weakness or numbness of the face, arm, or leg
- loss of speech or trouble speaking or understanding speech
- dimness or loss of vision, particularly in only one eye or half of both eyes
- sudden onset of blurred or double vision
- unexplained dizziness
- sudden onset of unsteadiness, lack of coordination, falling, or difficulty walking
- sudden excruciating headache
- recent change in personality or mental abilities, including memory loss.

OTHER MEDICAL CONDITIONS BESIDES STROKE

Approximately 50 to 70 percent of people who have a stroke or a recurrence have high blood pressure. A significant number have heart conditions, diabetes, and numerous other medical conditions, particularly those related to aging. Each year, about 1 percent of people between ages 65 and 74 have a stroke. About 5 to 8 percent of people in that age group who have a "ministroke" go on to have a fuller stroke.

In addition to the warning signs and symptoms of stroke, family members need to know the symptoms that signal an emergency for other existing medical conditions. A good way to begin is for family members to talk with the primary-care physician about the specific symptoms and signs of an emergency medical condition or a combination of medical conditions occurring at the same time. You will also want to learn about the possible reactions from prescribed medications that need to be reported and the kinds of pain related to the condition that may be experienced. If there has been surgery, you definitely will want to know about the signs and symptoms that need to be reported to your doctor immediately.

HOW FAMILY MEMBERS CAN HELP IN AN EMERGENCY

- Focus on what you realistically can do.
- Although you may be frightened, do everything in a steady and reassuring manner. The person with the problem usually is conscious, can see your facial expression, and will react if you have panic in your eyes or in your voice.

- Your grasp of the situation may be better than that of the person who is experiencing the emergency. If you suspect an emergency, get help *immediately* even if your family member wants to wait.
- Trust your ability to handle priorities.
- Tell yourself that you can't panic.
- Reassure yourself that you are doing your best and you *will* be able to help.

SOME EMERGENCY SAFEGUARDS

The Rusk Institute rehabilitation team recommends these safeguards to family members.

- **Be able to identify the early signs of a stroke or other emergency.** If a family member has recently undergone surgery or a medical procedure, and has—in addition to stroke—high blood pressure, diabetes, or a heart condition (with a valve replacement and/or a pacemaker), ask your doctor for the warning signs you need to know for these medical conditions.
- **Know what to do in an emergency.** Write down the steps you need to follow in an emergency that you have learned about from the doctor.
- **Know about the hospitals nearest your home with 24-hour emergency care.**
- **Keep a list of emergency rescue numbers next to the telephone and carry a copy with you.** In addition, make sure that everyone in the family knows where the numbers are kept. (A chart on page 260 offers a prototype for making your own list.) Also carry a copy of the telephone numbers of people to call in an emergency in your wallet or purse.

- **Carry a list of all your medications with you.** In addition, make sure that everyone in the family carries an up-to-date list of medications for emergency medical personnel to refer to.
- **Act immediately.** If your family member is experiencing the signs of a stroke or heart attack, or any other pronounced symptoms of pain or debility, make every effort to reach the doctor—but do not delay getting to the hospital.
- **Expect a "denial" from your family member.** It's normal for someone to deny the possibility of something as serious as a stroke because they are frightened. *Don't let this stop you.* Take prompt action anyway. Most people wait close to two hours before calling the doctor or getting to the hospital for the medical care they need.
- **Make every effort to remain reassuring.** After Emergency Medical Service (EMS) has been called and you are waiting for help to arrive, make every effort to remain calm and reassuring. Make the person comfortable by loosening clothing, such as by opening a collar or a belt. It may be better for the person to be sitting rather than lying down, in case vomiting occurs. Except for some water, it is best not to allow the person to drink anything.
- **Learn about Medic Alert.** This organization can assist you in an emergency by giving information to the Emergency Medical Service and the hospital. Medic Alert is more fully described later in this chapter.

CALLING THE EMERGENCY MEDICAL SERVICE (EMS)

You can dial 911 in an emergency and get help in more than 50 percent of the country, according to the American Red Cross. By dialing 911, you can activate the Emergency Medical Service (EMS), the fire department, and the police. In many parts of the country, you can reach 911 without inserting a coin in a pay phone. If you are uncertain of the phone number for emergency medical services when in the midst of an emergency, dial "0" and the operator will connect you to them.

Some communities do not have a 911-emergency telephone system. The local telephone books provide a listing of emergency services within those communities. It is very important to have this number handy.

Here is the recommended procedure for contacting EMS:

- **You activate the emergency medical service by dialing the number in your community.** When you report that you suspect a medical emergency, you will be connected to an emergency medical service dispatcher who will ask you your address.
- **Give the exact location of where you are.** If you are at home, give your street address, the cross streets, and the number of your house. If it's an apartment house or multifamily dwelling, be sure to give the apartment number, floor, or other location. If the building has more than one entrance or elevator, you can save a few minutes by specifying detailed information. If you are at work, give the building, the floor, and any other details about how to find you.
- **Give your name and the telephone number from which you are calling.**
- **Make sure that the emergency medical service dispatcher has the complete address—and the**

exact location—and your phone number. Let the
emergency medical service dispatcher hang up first.
* **If the emergency occurs at night, turn on an outside light.** If possible, send someone out to watch for
  the emergency medical service in order to direct the
  rescue personnel. Usually at least two emergency
  medical service personnel will arrive with equipment.
* **Be prepared to give the emergency medical service technicians, as well as the doctors in the hospital, the names of all prescribed medications,
  details of the physical condition of the stricken
  person, and the name and telephone number of
  the person's doctor.**

How Your Doctor Can Help in an Emergency

Call your doctor—even if you know it's just a number for
the answering service. The doctor's telephone answering
service can locate him or her, or they can contact the
doctor covering the practice. Even if it is a weekend or
after hours, don't assume that the doctor will be unavail-
able in an emergency. Notify the doctor, but if you suspect
that you or someone you know is having a stroke, heart
attack, or other medical emergency, get to the hospital
without delay. This is especially important if the person
previously had a stroke or heart attack.

* **Review the various procedures with your doctor,
  before an emergency occurs.** When you next see
  your doctor, ask what to do when you need to get to
  the hospital or call the emergency medical service
  without waiting for the doctor's return call. Find out

the location of the hospital nearest to your home that has 24-hour emergency service, as well as one near where you work. Perhaps your doctor can help you work out an emergency plan.

- **Ask your doctor which symptoms indicate an emergency.** Find out the specific signs that indicate an emergency, and collect information you and your family need to give the emergency medical service and the hospital.

- **Ask your doctor for other safeguards you should consider.** If you are alone for long periods of time, find out if your doctor recommends that you consider a personal response system, such as Medic Alert, so you can quickly and directly alert the emergency medical system. (For information about personal security systems, see page 104 later in this chapter.)

WHERE YOU CAN LEARN CARDIOPULMONARY RESUSCITATION (CPR) AND FIRST AID

Local chapters of the American Red Cross and many Ys and community centers offer a nine-hour hands-on course in CPR that allows you to learn and practice your skills on a specially designed mannequin, with supervision from an instructor. Generally, the course is given either in one day or in three-hour sessions one day a week for three weeks. Your local chapter of the American Heart Association can refer you to a class in your community.

EMERGENCY MEDICAL IDENTIFICATION

Five million Americans are treated in hospital emergency rooms every year. A doctor you've probably never met before will have only a few minutes to make important decisions about the care you need. That doctor in the hospital must have accurate information immediately about your medical condition, which medications you take, and which you are allergic to.

Emergency medical professions recommend the following:

- Wear a universally recognized emblem around the wrist or neck that can be custom-engraved with your personal medical conditions.
- Look for a service that gives its medical staff 24-hour telephone access to your computerized medical records.
- Be sure the service can store and quickly retrieve your vital medical information plus the telephone numbers of your doctors and two people you designate to be called in an emergency.
- Don't rely on carrying only a wallet card. Emergency personnel often don't have time or are not allowed to search your purse or wallet. They are trained to look for an alerting emblem on your wrist or neck. Once you put on an emergency medical identification bracelet or neck chain, don't take it off. It could save your life.

Medic Alert Foundation

Medic Alert Foundation International provides emergency medical information quickly and accurately to emergency personnel via a 24-hour toll-free telephone hotline. The organization maintains computerized records on an individual's medical conditions, medications, and the telephone numbers of your doctor and two people you have designated to be called in case of an emergency.

Medic Alert also maintains an international implant registry for all types of implants, including heart valve prosthesis and pacemakers. A newsletter and updates of recalls and new research are sent to members, doctors, and hospitals.

A basic lifetime membership is only $35 and is a tax-deductible medical expense. The fee includes emergency hotline service, a custom-engraved stainless-steel wrist or neck emblem with chain attached (sterling and gold-plated emblems are slightly more expensive), and a wallet card copy of all computerized information. Some men and women have the words *stroke/memory impaired*, as well as the name of a person to notify in case of an emergency, printed on their bracelet or necklace if they have a tendency to get lost while on their own.

For more details, write Medic Alert Foundation, Turlock, California 95381-1009, or call 1-800-ID-ALERT. Most pharmacies have Medic Alert enrollment forms that you can fill in and mail.

PERSONAL ALERT EMERGENCY RESPONSE SYSTEMS

An estimated half a million Americans subscribe to private systems that provide access to emergency medical services. Chances are that you've seen their dramatic advertisements on television.

The system itself consists of a small push-button device, typically worn comfortably around the neck or carried in a pocket. It can be activated by a hand squeeze to transmit a signal to a monitoring center through a transmitter unit attached to the telephone. An operator will try calling the user back when the signal is received. If no one answers or if someone answers and reports that a crisis exists, a call is placed to the Emergency Medical Service and the doctor.

These home-alert systems go by a variety of names such as Lifeline, Lifewatch, Lifecall, and other similarly descriptive terms. Lifeline, the first such system available to the public, reports that they have about one-hundred thousand subscribers.

Costs for the subscriber's initial equipment for the many systems available throughout the country vary anywhere from $300 to $900, with monthly service costs generally ranging from $10 to $20. To find out what systems are available in your area, call the hospital discharge office and the Agency on Aging in your area. Be sure to investigate thoroughly any system you may consider buying for its effectiveness as well as its total cost—which includes monthly service charges plus the rental or purchase price for the home-based equipment. Contact the Better Business Bureau to see if they have had any complaints about the particular company you're considering.

The National Rehabilitation Information Center (1-800-346-2742) will send you a listing of most of the personal security systems available.

DRIVING SAFELY

In his thirty years as a driving instructor at the Rusk Institute, Jiri Sipajlo has trained thousands of drivers with disabilities, including people who have had a stroke. "Most of us take for granted the ability and the need to get around," he says; and he agrees that for someone with a physical disability who can no longer use the public transportation system in the usual way, the need to drive to work and to maintain independence is essential.

Although driving after a stroke is not for everyone, many who thought they would not drive again are doing so successfully, after passing an evaluation and, if necessary, taking a driver's training course. When asked how many driving lessons on average a person generally needs after a stroke, Sipaljo says, "I can't generalize with an answer because it depends entirely on the individual and the degree of involvement of the disability. It is conceivable that I can do the evaluation and everything can be completed for some drivers within three hours, while others may require more extensive training."

Each state varies in its requirements for drivers who have had a stroke. To learn the procedure for reporting a disability in your particular state, you should call the local motor vehicle department. "Although states have different laws, common sense will tell you that if you've lost the use of a hand or an arm, a foot or a leg, or if you're prone to fainting, dizzy spells, seizures, convulsions, or loss of consciousness, pertinent details about current and past medical conditions should be reported before driving again," he says. In some states, the motor vehicle department may require a letter from a physician stating that it is safe for a person to drive on a public highway, but the physician will not be able to know this until a person is evaluated by a qualified instructor of an approved program for drivers with disabilities. The driving instructor, in turn, reports to the physician whether the driver can drive or should return for another evaluation at a later date.

"Even if the law doesn't require a driving evaluation, it makes sense to have a qualified instructor rate your driving ability," says Sipaljo. In order to drive again after a stroke, he believes that it helps to have training in order to build confidence and motivation.

The Automobile Association of America (AAA) publishes the "Handicapped Driver's Mobility Guide," which lists the agencies, schools, and individuals in each state who are qualified and certified to teach and evaluate drivers with disabilities. It also lists companies that modify cars and vans to meet individual needs. The guide is available from your local AAA for $5.95.

For example, when the right side of the body is affected after a stroke, the driver then drives with the left side of the body using a steering knob on the left side of the steering wheel at about the eight o'clock position. A left-side accelerator extension device, which is mounted on the floor, enables the driver to operate the gas and the brake with the left foot.

If the driver has weakness of the left side, a steering knob is mounted on the steering wheel at about four o'clock. The exact placement of the knob depends on the design of the wheel, the presence of air bags, and the spokes of the steering wheel. For this driver, a right-handed directional signal extension will be needed. Since today's cars have high and low beams, windshield wipers, and other features combined in the directional signal, the driver with left-side involvement needs to pull over to the side of the road when it is about to rain—stop the car—and then activate the windshield wipers.

All drivers need to drive five cars. When driving in heavy traffic, you have to drive five cars: your own car, the car ahead of you, the car behind you, and the two cars on either side of you. Among other things, the instructor is evaluating the driver's judgment in interpreting signs and symbols, in perceiving the traffic flow, and what other people are trying to do. A driver who is overly careful can be just as dangerous as one who drives at excessive speeds.

Sipajlo says that extensive instruction may be needed to retrain driving skills and to restore confidence in the ability to drive. Are the driver's judgment, sense of timing, perception, and navigation intact? The instructor is evaluating all these factors, as well as the driver's confidence in driving proficiently and with care. The ultimate goal is individual mobility with competence and safety.

DR. A. J. BERMAN*, NEUROSURGEON

Everybody's different and every stroke is different. It can involve a small blood vessel or a larger blood vessel—which means that more blood tissue was affected. In my position as a doctor, it's not very pleasant to know all that I know. However, I look at it from another point of view: after what I've been through, I'm very lucky to be recovering so well now. So I tend to see all this on the positive side.

I still have some weakness on the left side and double vision, so I continue going for rehabilitation. I go three times a week and sometimes even four times a week. And they say that I'm doing very well. I'm walking unaided, and some scientist friends of mine have put together a pair of glasses for me to correct the double vision, which means that I can read and I can watch TV and go to the movies.

> **"I've found that the fatigue connected with this condition is immense."**

I've found that the fatigue connected with this condition is immense. They say it's not uncommon to have this fatigue for a minimum of six months, but I just wasn't prepared for the extent of it. I used to be in the operating room by eight in the morning, and some nights I wouldn't get home until 11:00. I put in very long days, and I never used to sit still for a moment. Now, as soon as I come back from the rehabilitation—I'm home by 4:00 or 5:00 P.M.—I'm so tired that I'm ready to go to bed. And I could stay asleep until eight or nine o'clock the next morning.

My stamina is the worst, and how much more I used to

---

* This is a pseudonym.

have I never realized as a practicing neurosurgeon. I do a lot of neurosurgery, as well as an awful lot of work under the microscope—particularly with my experimental work. Whenever people ask me, 'Well, aren't you depressed since you were such an active person?' As a matter of fact, I think it hasn't been that easy accepting the need to slow down.

I had surgery last December, and I left the rehabilitation center in March, and I've been an outpatient there since. When they said I had a stroke on the left side, and that I had a weakness, I thought that even when I was at the rehabilitation center my weakness had recovered. But to my surprise, when I looked at my handwriting, and saw it wasn't as usual, I realized I still have some weakness. I can still move all my fingers and can do everything I need to so it won't interfere with my work. I'm already back to doing what I normally have to do. I just need to get a little practice at the hand-to-eye coordination, and I know I'll be able to do it soon.

Chapter Four

A Family Endeavor

People must help one another, it is nature's law.

—JEAN DE LA FONTAINE

WHAT MAY BE NEEDED

"It's not a question of *will* a stroke change your life, but *how* it changes it," says Michael Ajamian, who had a stroke after bypass surgery at age forty-four.

"A pitcher who pitches a no-hitter couldn't win without the help of the other eight players on the team," says Michael Ajamian. "My team is anyone who works with me in my recovery: my doctors and therapists, my family and friends, and paid helpers. I need them all to make it."

A stroke wasn't the only problem Ajamian had to face. "You put up with a dozen other major disappointments. Your employer isn't sure he wants you back, and the insurance company cuts off your coverage for therapy." Ajamian strongly suggests you find out exactly what your rights are from your employer, the insurance company, and anyone else you have to deal with in the current situation.

Six months into his rehabilitation program, Ajamian received a letter from his insurance company stating that his coverage for physical, occupational, and speech therapy had run out. His therapists felt there was more work to be done, but there wasn't a thing he or they could do about it. For a while, depression immobilized him. Then he got angry. "*I'm* the one who decides when I'm through working on getting well again. I was far from finished trying, and that's where my wife, kids, my parents, and aunt made the difference. We started what we jokingly called Ajamian University!

"There obviously is more that can and needs to be done beyond the work with a therapist," says Ajamian. "Physical, occupational, and speech therapy take place two or more times a week, forty-five minutes or less, and last several months for most people. No matter what puts an end to the formal therapy—the insurance runs out or rehab discharges you—it stands to reason you have to continue to work after therapy stops. That's your only ticket to get back some purpose in life after a stroke that hits you everywhere you live," he says.

Because his father and an uncle had had strokes and the family includes a doctor and three nurses, Ajamian felt confident that he would receive good medical care. Equally important to him was continuing the work of the physical, occupational, and speech therapists on his own or with therapists he paid for himself. To rebuild muscle tone and increase stamina after therapy ended he did his range-of-motion exercises at home, chores around the house, and joined a senior-citizen exercise program at a nearby Y. At first, fatigue overwhelmed him and he thought he might have to stop going to the class—but his need for structure kept him going. "Before the Y, I'd wake up in the morning with no place to go," he says. "The more I stayed home, the less confidence I had about going out, getting on a bus, and going somewhere." He felt the support of the people in his class, who "adopted" him and restored his self-esteem. "I had fifteen grandmothers, and it was the best medicine."

Before his stroke, Ajamian had bought a new car. Afterward, he wondered if he would be able to drive again. His wife located a driving instructor, and in two months he passed the driving test. The instructor recommended that he have a knob installed on the wheel to make it easier to turn. Driving restored his sense of independence. About a year after his stroke, Ajamian was able not only to return to work but also to drive himself there as well. He considered himself a very lucky man.

Each family has its own priorities and goals, and ultimately they decide what their needs are and how they will go about meeting them. Among the many factors a family may want to consider is: How intact are the abilities of their loved one with regard to moving about, communicating, comprehending, coping emotionally, and assuming responsibilities? And beyond that, what is the potential for their recovery?

After such an evaluation, each family member can decide what they are able to do to help, as well as the extent of the financial support they can give. If a caregiving member also has a job and is not at home during the day, or for other reasons is unable to provide care, a paid helper may be needed, and the family must decide if they can afford this service.

In general, families should review their financial resources. For example, does their insurance plan provide for good quality medical care? Is the insurance coverage sufficient to provide the physical, occupational, and speech therapies needed? If not, will there be enough money from other sources to cover ongoing therapy? Is there enough money to cover living expenses now and for the future? Are there changes necessary to ensure financial security?

Accessibility factors and the general safety of the home should be considered, with potential hazards eliminated to prevent falls and other accidents from occurring. If the layout needs improvement, can it be adapted so the bathroom, kitchen, and stairs pose no problems to a wheelchair user? Or the family might instead consider moving because of insurmountable architectural barriers, or to better their financial situation. When a family member who has had a stroke lives alone, alternative living arrangements may need to be explored. To remain living at home, it may be wise to rent out space to a boarder, for both financial and emotional reasons. Moving in with adult children or other relatives may be a solution.

Does the nearby transportation system provide convenient access to disabled passengers? Is it reasonable to expect that the family member who had a stroke will return to work—either at the old job or something new? And if the latter case is true, would vocational training make it possible to work at a new job or in the same job with some modifications. If the partner who worked outside the home must now remain at home, can the other partner go to work? If so, who will assume the household responsibilities?

In order to garner help in resolving many of these issues, family members and others who are planning home care and rehabilitation need the combined input and evaluation from the doctor, physical therapists, occupational therapists, speech therapists, and social workers. Examining the problems and challenges ahead from the vantage point of their training, professionals can help identify for the family both the deficits of the loved one who has had a stroke and the strengths and abilities on which to build. They can give the family a fuller understanding of its vital role in caring for and restoring their loved one to health.

Another valuable source of information is provided by men and women who have had a stroke and their families. We asked some of them how they made the transition from the hospital back to the home. We asked family members, "How do you help a loved one become self-sufficient and still maintain a life of your own? Their shared experiences, suggestions, and advice comprise this chapter.

WHAT FAMILIES CAN DO

First make a chart, such as the one on the page that follows, so that you may plan for each type of need and then arrange a time for the appropriate person, service, organization, or supplier to cover it. Leave space in each section for new items and other changes. Don't try to cram everything onto one sheet. You may want to use a loose-leaf notebook so that you can revise the chart after the work starts.

Suggestions for Families

- **The more you know, the more effective you can be.** The more you learn and understand about stroke, the effects it's had, and what you can expect, the more control you may have over the recovery process. Reading booklets and other pertinent publications plus talking to the doctor, therapists, and other people who have had a stroke are just a few of the ways to make yourself more knowledgeable and aid you in the ability to make informed decisions.

- **Be an active participant in the medical care of your loved one.** When it comes to medical care, remember that you're buying a service, so always think of yourself as a customer. Keep asking questions of the doctors, therapists, psychologists, social workers, and anyone else involved in your loved one's care *until you get the information you need*. Families need to find professionals in whom they have confidence.

  Medical care is the most personal service you can receive as a consumer. It's difficult to remember that the money is in *your* pocket, especially at times when you're most vulnerable. Even if the service is covered by insurance, you are the one who decides who's going to get what. (*No matter who is actually paying the bills, it's essentially still your money.*) As a consumer, you are entitled to your money's worth. As with any service you pay for, you have certain defined rights, and the more you know, the better you will be protected.

Help Needed

Type	Provided by Family or Friends	Provided by Personal-Care Aide	Provided by Other	No. of Days
Personal Care				
Grooming				
Bathing				
Dressing				
Eating				
Meal preparation				
Medications				
Assistance with physical therapy				
Transportation				
Accompanying to doctor, therapists, shopping				
Other _____				
Household				
Housekeeping				
Laundry				

Shopping
Banking
Bill paying
Other _____

Nursing Care
Postoperative care
Injections
Enteral feedings and
  hyperalimentation
Incontinence training
Other _____

Therapy
Physical therapy
Occupational therapy
Speech therapy
Cognition therapy

Help Needed (Continued)

TYPE	PROVIDED BY FAMILY OR FRIENDS	PROVIDED BY PERSONAL-CARE AIDE	PROVIDED BY OTHER	NO. OF DAYS
Psychological counseling				
Neuropsychological counseling				
Sexuality counseling				
Other _____				
Community Services				
Home health agencies				
Transportation service				
Meals-on-Wheels				
Adult day care				
Senior center				
Telephone reassurance				
Friendly Visitor Program				
Religious-affiliated services				
Agencies on aging				
Community agencies and programs				

Chore services				
Independent living centers				
Other _____				
Adaptive Equipment for Self-Sufficiency				
Eating utensils				
Telephone				
Television/closed captioning				
Computer				
Bathtub chair				
Wheelchair/transfer board				
Other _____				

You can be assertive while still being reasonable and polite. In evaluating professionals, you need to ask yourself if the doctor or therapist is capable, caring, and someone you trust. A professional may be capable but may not be right for you, and only you can know that.

- **Family members are partners in the recovery.** Strike a balance between pushing and coddling. Some families hold the belief that if their loved one works harder, they will achieve more; when in reality, most people are already putting forth their best efforts. Other families tend to overprotect and do too much for the loved one who is recovering from a stroke, while claiming that it's in their best interest to take it slowly. It's important to maintain a balance between these two extremes when continuing the valuable therapy work at home. Family members shouldn't feel as if they're in school; neither should they feel they're once again in the hospital.

- **Divide the responsibilities among everyone in the family.** Home care is often all-consuming and can become the entire focus of a family's life. In order for a primary caregiving family member to get enough rest and a chance to renew, families find it best to include everyone, including grandchildren, who can do shopping and run errands. In sharing responsibilities, individuals can do different tasks in accordance with their other time demands and their usual roles within the family. For example, the family member who goes out to work each day may find it easier to be the one to provide financial help and take care of outside chores like shopping and going to the bank. The person who is traditionally responsible for running the household and has little or no outside employment may be the one to handle the bills and correspondence and do the driving to and from therapy and doctor's appointments.

- **Families need to learn to communicate in new ways.** When a family member has aphasia and becomes frustrated finding the exact words to express themselves, don't be critical, and allow them time before jumping in to help. Many families find that familiar voices and surroundings and structured, repetitive routines are helpful, as are the use of short sentences and both verbal and non-verbal cuing. Choose a quiet, relaxed time, without distracting background noise, to share the day's events. Balance the daily routine by following stimulating activities with a quiet time, but not in such a manner that the family member is isolated. Include your family member in conversations and decisions so that the pattern of inclusion becomes habitual.

- **Learn ways to help reduce the mental fatigue of your loved one.** Notice the periods of peak alertness, and schedule important activities during these times. Try brief periods of 5 to 10 minutes of focused attention, interspersed with rest periods. Later on, the number and length of the activity times can be increased. Provide enough to interest and stimulate, but not so much that it overwhelms or confuses. Be patient and repeat instructions, if necessary. Draw upon special personal interests to stimulate activity without mental fatigue, such as preparing a favorite snack, playing a game, and looking at a magazine.

- **Create an environment that will increase attention and concentration.** Turn off the television or radio, and try to eliminate other background noises. Stand so that your face can be seen. Before giving instructions, make sure that you have the person's attention. When there is a loss of interest because the person's concentration is diffusing, gently touch your loved one. Instead of repeating the instructions, just say the person's name or something simple and reassuring. If this doesn't regain the person's focus, go on to something else. Fatigue interferes with concentration, so it's best to choose times when someone is well rested.

- **Be aware of your own energy levels.** You are human and do not have unlimited physical and psychological energies. When you find that you are becoming tired or irritated, take a break. You're entitled to take time off—it's in everyone's best interest. Don't forget to schedule juice breaks and other sustenance for yourself and others in the family.
- **Families may be afraid of expressing real feelings.** Whether you are a wife, husband, an adult daughter or son, you may be afraid to express your real feelings for fear it will upset your loved one and interfere with his or her recovery. Family members need to talk about the changes that have taken place in their lives, especially when the family feels overburdened. It helps to discuss any resentments with one another, as well as with other families who have had similar experiences. This way, problems are more easily identified, and the family can more easily uncover solutions when they know they are not alone. In fact, expressing feelings authentically and appropriately, instead of storing them up or allowing them to simmer, helps to reestablish a balance in the family relationship.
- **A role reversal takes getting used to.** If the partner who was the wage earner must now remain at home while the other partner becomes the wage earner, the new roles will require some adjustment. Each of you must cooperate and adapt to the different responsibilities. Talking with other family members who have undergone similar experiences can help. Stroke clubs are good places to learn about what has worked for others.
- **Family members are welcome at stroke club meetings.** "There's nothing like being with people

who are experiencing something that you are," says a member of a stroke club for caregivers. Many stroke clubs have meetings for caregiving family members. Meetings are open to men and women who have had a stroke, their families, and anyone else who is interested. When a person who has had a stroke doesn't want to go to a meeting, family members can still attend, learn from the experience, and discuss the meeting when they return home.

- **Counseling often gives the family a new perspective.** Psychologists, particularly those who are experienced in working with poststroke emotional effects, can tell families how they can help. Because stroke is a medical crisis, the entire family is affected. It therefore is essential that families have a better understanding of what they are experiencing and feeling. Psychological counseling often gives families a perspective they would not otherwise have. Neuropsychologists are trained and experienced in working with family members after the stroke of a loved one. An evaluation of personality, motivation, coping abilities, degree of agitation, decision-making powers, impulsivity factors, and emotional reactions to disability can help the entire family. (More about coping with the emotional aspects of stroke can be found in Chapter Six, "Lifelong Learning," page 167.)
- **The encouragement of friends makes a difference.** Most friends rally 'round when there is an illness. Frequently, however, because of their own fear of illness, some friends might withdraw. If you and your family value the friendship, try to talk it out together with any valued friend who you feel may be pulling away.
- **A sense of humor helps diffuse stressful times, as can planning for recreational events.** A family member says, "I'm not saying we're the happiest

family on the block, but when we *can* laugh about
something, we don't let it pass us by." Humor can
provide wonderful relief from coping with daily frus-
trations and stress. The planning and experience
of family outings and other pleasurable events is
also a stress-reducing activity; and, of course, the
event itself can be fondly recalled after the actual
experience.

- **Families have valuable information for therapists.** Families know their loved one best and know
  their aspirations, priorities, goals, skills, and hob-
  bies. Therapists can incorporate this information
  into the therapeutic work to motivate, encourage,
  and make the experience more meaningful.
- **Ask the therapists for concrete ways that family
  members can continue their work in your home.**
  From the therapists you can learn about exercises,
  workbooks, games, computer software, and other
  services, all of which will help build muscle tone and
  stamina, enhance memory, and improve communication. (For a list of sources for information, workbooks, and computer software, see pages 231–239 in
  Chapter Seven, "Information, Services, and Products.")
- **Learn about the services in your community that
  may augment the options for home care and the
  recovery process.** The more families know about
  the services in their community, the more likely they
  are to enlist other people to help. A good starting
  point is the section (often on blue pages) of the telephone book that lists government agencies. In the
  Yellow Pages, you will find the kinds of organizations
  you are seeking under "Social and Human Services."
  In addition, a telephone company or other organization in your community may publish a directory that
  lists support services.

- **Have an informal, flexible, but structured schedule.** Everyone benefits from planning ahead. Break down tasks into their basic components and allow time to complete them. If clothes are laid out and the table set for breakfast the night before, it saves repeated trips and energy and encourages a sense of independence. (For specific strategies, see Chapter Two, "Recovering at Home," page 49). Try to notice the peak times of energy and awareness, and plan activities for those times. Leave enough time for rest after eating, bathing, dressing, and any other activities that are tiring. A schedule that is built on repetition of activities interspersed with rest is most likely to be successful for the loved one who has had a stroke.

- **Physical and occupational therapists can teach family members how to assist without injuring themselves.** By learning from the appropriate therapists how to assist in transfers, lifting, and readjusting positions, you can avoid potential accidents and injury. Books for nurse's aides (available from your local library) are useful because they have instructions and illustrations for safe and efficient ways to manage transfers and other tasks that require proper body mechanics. One or two home nursing visits can give you an assessment of the home-care needs and the answers to many of your questions. (Transferring tips are on page 66.)

- **If you don't take care of yourself, who will?** Hands-on, round-the-clock caregiving is all-consuming. You need time off, especially if you are the only family member involved in care. Consider getting help for shopping and other chores from a part-time personal-care aide, a housekeeper, or a student. If you set up a specific schedule, you are more likely to find a helper. You may want to post a notice

or look at the listings on the bulletin boards in houses
of worship, supermarkets, senior citizen centers, and
libraries. Independent living centers usually have
listings of personal-care aides and companions. Area
agencies on aging may be able to recommend community organizations or individual helpers.

• **Have an emergency plan ready that everyone in
  the family knows.** Everyone should know the signs
  and symptoms of an emergency, the steps to take,
  and the telephone numbers to call. This is important
  in every family, but it's essential in the family with a
  person who has had a stroke, heart attack, or other
  medical problem. Your local chapter of the American
  Heart Association and the National Stroke Association (800-STROKES) have printed material about
  the warning signs of a stroke. The American Red
  Cross and Ys offer classes in cardiac pulmonary re-
  suscitation (CPR) and abdominal thrusts in case of
  choking.

ENERGY SAVERS FOR THE FAMILY

• **Shop by phone and mail.** These days, you can order
  just about anything you want by phone or mail and
  have it delivered in a reasonable period of time. Overnight delivery is available from many mail-order
  companies, usually for an extra charge. Shop at
  stores that offer delivery services so you needn't
  carry heavy packages. Food, drugs, and other items
  can be delivered within minutes from local stores.
  You can order complete meals from many restau-
  rants, not just pizza joints.

• **Hire an errand runner.** Sometimes it's easier to hire
  someone for one day a week to run all your errands,

rather than doing them yourself. High school and college students can go shopping, do chores, as well as serve as companions on outings and visits to the doctor. Bulletin boards in supermarkets, churches, temples, libraries, and colleges are good places to post a job-opportunity notice.

- **Start your day the night before.** Prepare your "To Do List" for each day, keeping in mind you may want to revise your list in response to how you are feeling, your energy level, and other changeable priorities. Be prepared to renegotiate deadlines with yourself.
- **Sit rather than stand.** While bathing, brushing your teeth, washing dishes, and other activities, it is usually better to sit instead of leaning on the counter or standing. Sit on a stool or folding chair you keep in the bathroom and kitchen. Use a lightweight tray table on wheels to save trips going back and forth from the kitchen countertop to the table.
- **Avoid rush hour traffic, if possible.** Schedule appointments to avoid peak hour traffic. If that's not possible, you should practice relaxation breathing and allow for extra time to avoid the anxiety of rushing.
- **Each doctor's office is different, so plan your appointments accordingly.** Some doctors start at 7 A.M., and that may be much too early for you, particularly since you must allow enough time to dress and travel. For some, the last appointment is actually better because the doctor may be able to give you more time and answer your questions in a more leisurely way. Ask the receptionist or nurse about the doctor's schedule. Some doctors start their days at the hospital, so their offices are jammed by the time they arrive for their first appointments.
- **Don't lift or push anything heavy.** Try to push or slide objects rather than lifting them. When you do have to carry something, remember to exhale both

when you pick it up and during times of unusual exertion.

- **Cook for more than one meal at a time.** When preparing meals, refrigerate or freeze individual portions for future use.
- **Organize the things you use most often.** In both your house and workplace, have the things you use most often close at hand, so that you don't have to reach or bend for them.
- **Schedule a breather for yourself.** Either at home or at work, take time out to relax by closing your eyes and putting your feet up. If your work is especially stressful, arrange for leisure activities that are noncompetitive. Be wary of overscheduling yourself— take a day off!

HOME-CARE SERVICES

Some of the basic services that can be provided in the home include:

- medical and skilled nursing care
- therapies—physical, occupational, speech, respiratory, intravenous drug
- nutrition and dietary services
- hospice services
- medical equipment, including oxygen tanks, portable ventilators, and telephone devices for monitoring pacemakers.

Some agencies provide a wide range of services that include assistive devices such as walkers, wheelchairs and other equipment, and pharmaceutical and laboratory services. Personal-care services, including personal-care aides and other assistants, are nonmedical services that help with bathing, dressing, preparing meals, and other personal needs.

At the time of discharge from the hospital, your doctor may prescribe home-nursing visits, as well as physical and speech therapies. Often therapy begins at home, then continues with visits to the hospital or rehabilitation center.

Most hospital discharge planning offices can arrange for home-care visits of professionals through a home-care agency or an affiliate—if you request that they do so. About half of all hospitals have home-care agencies. Since most insurance companies require that the professional staff be from approved agencies, families need to make sure that the hospital agency checks out with the insurance requirements. If not, you may need to go further to find another agency.

A home-care nursing visit is likely to entail an assessment of the medical condition, monitor vital signs, and provide other care based on the doctor's orders. An integral part of a nursing visit is to educate the family by giving instructions and answering their questions about home care, medications, and any pain or discomfort.

If home visits are not prescribed, are limited, or not covered by insurance, the family may decide to have a personal-care aide help them at home in the early days after leaving the hospital. This is especially recommended if your loved one has had surgery or the primary caregiving family members are at work, have their own medical problems, or are elderly. If the person who has had a stroke lives alone, it may be a good idea to hire a personal-care aide or housekeeper who can shop, prepare, and serve meals. Some aides have their own cars or can drive the family car. This is especially helpful on visits to the doctors or other therapists, particularly when a family member is not available.

Even if it is on a part-time basis—and not covered by insurance—someone assisting can give family members a chance to rest and renew, or return to work. "Someone who is kind, caring, and capable is an essential ingredient of recovery—and every family's dream," says Bryna Marantz, whose husband, Art, had a stroke. "It gives the caregiver a much-needed chance for a break—to relax and rejuvenate, to leave the house for a few hours to do some other things that matter, or to return to work without worrying about leaving their loved one alone." Marantz has had the best experiences with several personal-care aides from one agency she swears by. She finds that you sense very quickly whether a personal-care aide, a physical therapist, or any other professional is going to be a part of the solution or otherwise.

Personal-care aides from agencies assist *only* the person they are assigned to care for. They are not expected to prepare meals or do laundry or chores for other members of the family. The law in most states does not permit an aide to dispense medications, to change sterile dressings, give injections, or draw blood for tests. A personal-care aide is supervised by a nurse and other professionals at the home-care agency.

Many families decide to recruit, train, and manage a personal-care aide *outside* of the auspices of an agency, although it may take considerable time to locate a person who is reliable, trustworthy, and pleasant. They often learn of someone who is available from a family member, friend, or neighbor. Another good place to ask is at a stroke club meeting, or while chatting with people in your doctor's office.

"Great health-care professionals don't just walk up to you. Finding them is an active process," says Tom Watson, who employs several aides on a part-time basis. "Someone who is good helps me by letting me do what *I* can do, and helps me to do what wears me out. That person gives me choices by saying 'How about this?' and 'What if . . . ?' so I'm still my own person."

Men and women who have had a stroke and employ personal-care aides, as well as the aides themselves, agree that the major factor in establishing long and mutually satisfying employer-employee relationships is respect for each other's rights.

The reasons that aides are fired often include lack of dependability, or the fact that they prove to be physically, psychologically, or emotionally incapable of performing the required duties, or they are unreasonably slow or lazy. They may be dishonest with their employer's work time, possessions, finances, medications, or food; or they may lack respect for their employer's right to privacy and confidentiality.

The reasons that personal-care aides quit include the fact that they were given an incomplete list of duties or unclear instructions when they were hired, and they become frustrated or resentful as unexpected duties are added; or they feel unappreciated, the working environment is unpleasant and irritating, or they are addressed in an abusive manner.

"Caring for someone is really a partnership of both people," asserts a woman who has worked for the last fifteen years as a personal-care attendant. "You both need to keep the golden rule in mind and treat each other the way you would like to be treated. You want to know that you're appreciated and spoken to in the same manner that others expect from you."

The majority of personal-care assistants come from the recommendations of family and friends. Many people also get helpers and other assistance from nonprofit organizations such as the more than 200 nonresidential

Independent Living Centers across the country. These
Centers are operated by disabled consumers who coordinate or provide direct services in their community. Most
Centers maintain a list of experienced personal-care
aides, psychological support services to families, and
peer support. To find an Independent Living Center near
you, call or write the Southern Tier Independence Center,
107 Chenango Street, Binghamton, NY 13901, phone:
(607) 724-2111.

INSURANCE COVERAGE FOR HOME CARE

Medicare and most insurance coverage is restricted to a
person who is both homebound and requires part-time or
"intermittent" skilled nursing care plus physical or speech
therapy prescribed by a doctor for a limited number of
visits. This rules out coverage for around-the-clock home-
nursing care, which is reimbursed only under very restricted circumstances.

Medicare and many insurance plans do not cover nonmedical personal care or homemaker services, prescribed drugs, meals delivered to the home, blood
transfusions, respiratory therapists, transportation services, or professional nutrition and dietary services.
Each employer-provided group health maintenance organization and private insurance plan has its own
unique benefits and constraints. Some plans do provide
for nursing visits, hospital outpatient services, therapeutic services, and pharmaceuticals.

Home-care services must be prescribed by the doctor,
be accompanied by a written care plan, and then be approved by your insurance company or agency. All home
care, including physical therapy and speech therapy, must

be supervised by a registered nurse from an approved agency.

Most home-care agencies require that you sign an agreement or contract before they provide you with services. A contract commits you to pay for the services or authorizes the agency to bill your insurance company or Medicare.

The services provided by home health-care agencies vary widely in cost, depending on the particular region of the country and on the agency itself. Costs are usually higher outside of large metropolitan areas and in outlying rural areas. Charges are usually figured on a per-visit basis, though in some instances the services are billed on an hourly basis. An individual paying out-of-pocket for nursing services can pay more than $100 per visit or less than $75, depending on the agency and the part of the country. Professional visits of physical and speech therapists, as well as home visits of social workers, generally run about the same as for nurses. Physical and speech therapists in private practice sometimes charge less than agencies.

The cost for the services of personal-care aides and homemakers vary, depending on the area of the country, the agency, and the responsibilities involved. Most agencies require a four-hour minimum for personal-care aides and set firm guidelines for their responsibilities.

Trying to understand the constraints on services placed by insurance coverage can be a confusing and frustrating experience. But there are people out there—like your insurance representative—who can make it less so. If your doctor prescribes home-nursing care or physical therapy and your insurance will cover the services, you can find the approved agencies in your community by asking the hospital social worker. Your insurance representative should be able to give you a list of the agencies to choose from, and you may call several of them directly in order to do a price comparison. Or your doctor may be able to recommend an approved agency. (For more details about locating home-care services in your community, see pages 224–228 in Chapter Seven, "Information, Services, and Products.")

A CLIENT HOME-CARE BILL OF RIGHTS

As a consumer, you have the right to:

* receive considerate and respectful care in your home at all times.
* participate in the development of your plan of care, including making sure you receive an explanation of any services proposed, with suggestions for alternative services that may be available in the community.
* receive complete written information on your plan of care including the name of the supervisor responsible for your services.
* refuse medications and counseling, or other services without fear of reprisal or discrimination.
* be fully informed of the consequences of all aspects of care, unless medically contraindicated, once the possible results of refusal of medical treatment, counseling, or other services are explained to you.
* privacy and confidentiality about your health, social, and financial circumstances, and what takes place in your home.
* expect that all communications and records will be treated confidentially.
* expect that all home-care personnel within the limits set by the plan of care will respond in good faith to your requests for assistance in the house.

- receive information on the agency's policies and procedures, including information on charges, qualifications of personnel, and on discontinuation of service.
- request a change of caregiver.
- participate in the plan for discontinuation of services.
- have home care as long as needed and available.
- have access upon request to all bills for service regardless of whether they are paid for out-of-pocket or through other sources of payment.
- receive nursing supervision of the homemaker/home health care aides, if medically related personal care is needed; and have such supervision be performed by a registered nurse.

(Reprinted by permission of the Foundation for Hospice and Home Care.)

CAROL LADERMAN, CHAIR, ANTHROPOLOGY DEPARTMENT, THE CITY UNIVERSITY OF NEW YORK

I think it was a very good thing that nobody told me, when I was really sick, that it was unlikely that I would ever get completely well again. So when I had that hemiplegia—it was impossible for me to move one side except a little bit—it never occurred to me that feeling and movement wouldn't come back. I just kept working on it, kept moving it a little, and it came back. And the same thing with the other signs—they took awhile, but I never thought that I wouldn't recover.

> "Sometimes you are in treatment with people who mean to do good, but they're just not good for you."

For people who have had a stroke, first and foremost it is important for them to know it is possible to recover. I think there is a danger in some people's attitudes—even some people who are involved in the field of rehabilitation—that once they know you have had this problem, it's very hard for them to believe you can ever be all right again. I had to break away from such attitudes in order to make the progress I have made. Sometimes you are in treatment with people who mean to do good, but they're just not good for you.

I've been considered a brave person throughout most of my life. And it just never occurred to me to worry that I wouldn't get all my faculties back. But it was rather awful not to be able to remember things. Like not remembering the names of people who had written books that I was very involved with for years. Some things came back little by little; some things I figured if I couldn't remember them, I knew where to look. At this point in my life, my memory has completely returned.

If you are a person who is going through what I've been through, I would tell you that you will get better. It will be fairly gradual, but it will keep on happening and probably within six months you will be better than you thought you would be before; within a year, you will be doing pretty well. I know some people who think that nobody gets all the way better. And maybe most don't; so I say to them, "What if I'm 90 percent better? Should I complain?"

In fact, I think I still have time to do even more recovering. My family helps. My husband is an artist, and also a professor, and he's been doing most of the cooking. He's pretty good—not as good as I used to be, but that's okay, because I don't want to cook. I cooked for forty years. He's so glad that I'm not dead! My kids are grown-up and they're good to me. They too were very shaken when I first had my stroke.

I went back to teaching even though people told me it would be hard. I got out of the hospital at the end of October, and I went back to school in January. Yes, it was very hard, but it was just the right thing for me to have done. If I hadn't done that, it would have taken me a much longer and harder time to recover. I was reelected at the end of the term as chair of my department for the next three years, so I guess I did the right thing.

Chapter Five

Taking Charge of Your Health

If we don't take good care of our bodies, where will we live?

—ANONYMOUS

INTRODUCTION

"No one knowingly sets out to have a stroke, high blood pressure, or a heart condition," asserts Michael Ajamian, whose stroke came after a bypass operation. "Many of the lifestyle choices which cause these conditions are learned from your family. Then throughout our lives, most of us continue to eat the familiar foods we ate while growing up. Those of us who are smokers often started as teenagers, and picked up the habit from following the example of family members. The amount of sports we did at home also usually influences how much activity we do later on in life. And our work habits and response to stress are also usually homegrown."

What we have learned in the last decade is that the three greatest risk factors for stroke—high blood pressure, heart disease, and diabetes—can be controlled or eliminated by modifying our diet, increasing our activity, not smoking, and not drinking excessively. Also significant, according to research, is that we sustain ourselves with people we care about and by a belief in our own ability to influence our well-being.

You can quickly gather from talking to your doctor that the power for healing resides with you and your continued willingness to substitute positive, healthful alternatives to your past unhealthy choices. You'll see a reduction in your serum cholesterol, high blood pressure, weight, and blood sugar (if you have diabetes) if you cut down significantly on fats, salt, and sugar, increase your activity, maintain a weight close to your optimum, throw out your cigarettes, and learn constructive ways to manage the stress of daily living.

At the Rusk Institute of Rehabilitation Medicine, we believe in the miraculous role you can play in your own wellness. By learning everything you can about your medical condition, the more apt you are to believe in your own ability to influence the outcome, set goals, relearn skills, and look for people who can assist you in all the best ways.

Some of the major steps most people need to take in order to deal with a medical condition resulting from stroke are:

- Learn which doctors and medical centers in your community specialize in your particular medical condition, so that you will receive the best possible medical care.
- Find out everything you can about your medical condition and the care you will need, so that you and your family can participate in the decisions that will need to be made.
- Reach out for all possible sources of support, including trusted professionals, your family and friends, and other people who have had a stroke.
- Gradually become as self-sufficient as possible, without necessarily doing everything by yourself.
- Understand your feelings of fear, anger, loss, sadness, and depression with the help of your family, friends, and appropriate professionals.

No Two Strokes Are Alike

When doctors say someone has had a stroke—or a cerebrovascular accident (CVA)—they are describing what has happened when the blood supply to, or within, the brain is suddenly disrupted.

In order to function properly, nerve cells within the brain must have a continuous supply of blood, oxygen, and glucose (or blood sugar). If this supply is impaired, parts of the brain may stop functioning temporarily; or, if the impairment is severe or lasts long enough, the brain cells die and permanent damage ensues. The movement and functioning of various parts of the body are controlled by these brain cells. The death of the brain cells is what produces the symptoms of the stroke.

About one-third of all strokes are preceded by a transient ischemic attack (TIA), commonly called a ministroke. The ministroke is a localized neurological problem caused by decreased blood flow which may last only a few minutes and be completely resolved within twenty-four hours.

There are three main causes of stroke. For one, a stroke may be caused by a cerebral thrombus, that is, a blood clot that forms in a brain artery, thereby blocking the flow of blood to the brain. Known as cerebral infarction or atherothrombic stroke, this condition accounts for about 70 percent of all strokes. Often preceded by ministrokes, they tend to occur at times when blood pressure is low—particularly at night during sleep or early in the morning before the start of the day's activities.

Another major cause of stroke is a cerebral embolus, which is a wandering blood clot. It originates in one part of the body, breaks loose, and travels through the bloodstream until it lodges in an artery in the brain or in a vessel leading to the brain. It is believed that most embolic strokes involve clots from the heart or the carotid arteries in the neck.

The third is a cerebral hemorrhage, which accounts for about 20 to 25 percent of all strokes. This entails the rupturing of a brain artery, which results in bleeding into the surrounding area of the brain.

A relatively small number of all strokes are caused by aneurysms. A cerebral aneurysm is the ballooning out of the wall of a blood vessel which forms at the point where the wall is weak. It may rupture and cause a hemorrhage.

It is also possible for clots to form in the pouch of the aneurysm, then to travel downstream, occlude a blood vessel, and cause a ministroke or stroke.

Other contributory causes of stroke include cardiac arrest and hematomas. A hematoma is an accumulation of blood that is the result of hemorrhage. It is usually caused by injury, but it may occur spontaneously, especially in the elderly.

Each stroke is unique. No two people who have brain injury are exactly alike. Each one reacts and recovers in a singular manner. Probably the best-known and most-common effect of stroke is paralysis or weakness of one side of the body; although the extent of the weakness or paralysis can vary from the entire side of the body to a slight weakness of an arm or leg. Hemiplegia—paralysis or weakness—usually occurs on the side of the body *opposite* the side of the brain where the injury occurred. Left hemiplegia involves damage to the right side of the brain and affects the left side of the body.

Approximately 20 percent of all people who have stroke have an impairment of communication abilities that is either temporary or permanent. Aphasia, the lack of ability to communicate, poses some of the most perplexing problems of brain injury and involves variously the ability to read, speak, recall, write, and grasp meaning, depending on the site and extent of the brain injury. These deficits may improve rapidly—within a few days or a week; but typically, recovery is a long process of months and even years.

After the acute phase of a ministroke or stroke has passed, emphasis is placed on medical treatment, rehabilitation, and educating people who have had a stroke in taking charge of their health. A primary goal is to teach them and their families how to prevent a recurrence by recognizing the warning signs of stroke and to seek immediate medical attention should this occur.

THE PURPOSE OF STROKE REHABILITATION

For some people, the goal is to mend, recuperate, and restore their bodies to a condition as healthy as it was before hospitalization. For others, the goal is to adapt to new ways of living that for a short period, or always, will be different from the way they lived before hospitalization.

In the hospital, rehabilitation after a stroke begins virtually at once, to prevent, minimize, recognize, and treat the potential impact of other complications. Other medical conditions can arise as a result of stroke and can limit an individual's ability to participate in his or her own recovery process. Preventing, identifying, and managing problems is very important. Some of these burdensome problems include shoulder dysfunction and pain, swallowing difficulties, pneumonia, seizures, incontinence, contractures, and pressure sores. In addition, it is estimated that as many as 67 percent of stroke survivors have high blood pressure, 47 percent have coronary artery disease, and 32 percent have diabetes; these conditions also must be monitored and controlled.

A major goal in stroke rehabilitation is maximum functional self-sufficiency, whether on one's own or with assistance. Working on an individualized basis, the professional team trains the stroke survivor in compensatory strategies, in methods to enhance and improve motor control in pursuing daily activities, and in communication skills.

According to Mike Morell, a physical therapist, the goals and purpose of stroke rehabilitation haven't changed very much in recent years. What has changed, however, is the amount of time Medicare and other insurance plans allow for their accomplishment.

"An opportunity exists for people who have had a stroke, and their families, to get involved in rehabilitation by asking questions and observe the therapies which can be continued at home," Morell says. "If it's financially feasible, pay for therapy yourself when the insurance runs out so you don't lose any of the gain you've already made; and, perhaps later, you can even exceed your expectations, or at the very least come back for an update."

To assist and support stroke survivors and their families in coping with and adapting to the physical, psychological, and communication disabilities that accompany it, a team of specialists from a variety of disciplines is necessary. These professionals often include the doctor, nurse, physical and occupational therapists, speech and language pathologists, neuropsychologist, social workers, orthotist, chaplain, vocational rehabilitation counselor, and recreation and art therapists.

Although many of these services are available in day and outpatient rehabilitation settings, many families do not utilize them. They often are unaware of their existence or are reluctant or unaccustomed to seeking psychological, marital, and sexuality counseling to resolve problems. Similarly, someone who would like to return to work may not know about the services a vocational rehabilitation counselor offers or where to find one.

After stroke rehabilitation, some people do better than expected, while others do not fare as well. For example, researchers in the Framingham Study (the oldest and largest comprehensive study on heart disease) found that 69 percent of stroke survivors become self-sufficient in their personal care, and 80 percent are able to walk after rehabilitation, depending on the severity of the stroke and on many other variable factors. Unfortunately, about two-thirds of the people in the Framingham Study reported decreases in both their ability to keep jobs and socialize outside of the home.

Many therapists have problems with the trend toward shorter hospital stays and the limits and constraints on insurance coverage for therapy. They try to include families in treatment early on in the rehabilitation process in order to prepare them for home-treatment programs after hospitalization. In day and outpatient rehabilitation settings, therapists collaborate with their clients and families in setting treatment goals to be carried out, at least in part, at home. Some therapists furnish printed materials and even make videos of exercises, and they encourage participation in stroke and aphasia clubs to gain support and avoid isolation.

Despite the odds, many people overcome formidable obstacles and achieve remarkable success. Invariably it takes an amalgam of personal motivation, strong coping style, physical fitness and good general health, support from family, good quality medical care, meaningful activity, financial security, and a solid network of friends and acquaintances.

"For me, recovering from my stroke has been to take charge of my life, but without doing everything myself," says Tom Watson. "I've been lucky to find some great people to teach me new ways to listen and talk and remember what was said. But the most important place my family and I have reached is a healthy—not resigned—acceptance of what has happened; so we've moved on from illness to see what else we want out of life."

SPECIFIC QUESTIONS FOR YOUR DOCTOR

While you are in the hospital or at your next appointment with your doctor outside the hospital you can learn more about your medical condition, the purpose of each medication, the ongoing treatment, and the changes in your condition that should be reported. If anything is unclear or confusing, ask to have it explained until you are certain you understand.

Here is a list of commonly asked questions of doctors who treat people who have had strokes. At various times during your recovery, you may want to reread this list to learn more about the areas of particular interest to you.

Your Medical Condition

- Can you describe my medical condition? What can I expect in terms of recovery?
- What do I and my family need to know about my medical condition, concurrent illnesses and side effects, pain, and warning signs of stroke? What do we need to know about managing high blood pressure, diabetes, heart disease, elevated cholesterol, or other medical conditions?
- What can you suggest for continued feelings of anxiety, depression, and other psychological and emotional reactions to stroke? When can I hope for some improvement? What do you suggest for others that brings them relief?
- What kind of pain and other symptoms should be reported to you?
- Which hospital do you recommend in case of an emergency? Which ambulance service do you recommend?
- Which activities must I avoid? For how long?
- When may I resume sexual activity? What do I need to know about the effect of my condition on sexual activity? If I experience problems, can you offer me support or recommend the services of other professionals?
- If I return to work, what do I need to know about modifying my work routine?

- Will you send a report and/or speak with my other doctors about my hospitalization, including details about my surgery, results of my tests and procedures, and the medications you have prescribed?

Exercise

- What physical therapy should I continue at home? Should I be doing range-of-motion exercises? If so, how frequently, and for what length of time?
- Should I be walking or doing other exercise? Are there any precautions I should take? Should I monitor my pulse during exercise? Why is checking my pulse and staying below my prescribed heart rate so important? (For more about setting exercise goals, see pages 200–201.)

Food

- What modifications do I need to make in my diet?
- Can you recommend programs that have helped others you treat? (For more about modifying diet and strategies to use, see pages 187–191.)

Medications

- What are the generic or brand names of each medication? What is each for, and what are the expected results?
- How much should be taken at one time? How often should I take it? When?
- How should it be taken? With food? On an empty stomach?

- How soon should the medication take effect? How long should I wait before calling you if it doesn't help?
- What are the foods, vitamins, and alcoholic beverages to be avoided?
- What are the over-the-counter pharmaceutical products that may not be used when taking the medication? Why?
- May the amount be doubled next time if one dose is missed?
- If I feel better, should I stop taking the medication?

Possible Side Effects

- What are the possible side effects or adverse reactions?
- What are the specific side effects that must be reported immediately?
- What are the possible psychological effects I may have from the medication?
- If I drive, is it safe to do so when taking any of my prescribed medications?
- Will the medication affect my pulse rate? What bearing might this have in monitoring my pulse when exercising?

GETTING THE BEST MEDICAL CARE

- **Have one doctor who consolidates all your health care.** Have a primary-care physician who coordinates your medications from each of the doctors who treat you.

- **Your family physician can refer you to a neurologist.** When considering a neurologist, consider a board-certified specialist who is on the staff of a medical center or hospital, preferably affiliated with a medical school. Board-certified neurologists usually use the initials F.A.C.N. after their names to signify membership as a Fellow of the American College of Neurology, a professional association whose members must be board certified. However, a board-certified neurologist may choose not to become a member of this association and still be fully qualified.
- **Ask your doctor to refer you to a neuropsychologist.** Experienced in the psychological and behavioral effects of stroke, a neuropsychologist can help families understand the psychological effects of stroke, offer coping strategies, and a new perspective that may be useful.
- **Check the doctor's credentials.** No matter where the recommendation comes from, you and your family can check a doctor's training, certification as a specialist, and membership in medical associations. Major libraries have the *American Medical Directory*, which has lists of all physicians and their credentials. To make sure that a doctor is certified by a group recognized by the American Board of Medical Specialties, call (800) 776-2378.
- **Work on establishing a partnership with your doctors.** The relationship with your doctors should be one in which you both talk and listen. Actively participate in all the decisions that are made about your treatment. If you have a conflict with your doctor or you can't work together, you may need to find another. Before changing doctors, try to resolve any conflict about your care.
- **Don't hesitate to get a second opinion.** Do not be inhibited by thinking that your doctor will be

offended if you consult another doctor for an opinion, particularly when a medical procedure or surgery has been recommended.

- **Give your dentist and other health-care professionals a list of all your medications.** If you have a
heart condition with a valve involvement, you need
to notify your doctor and dentist before you have a
dental procedure, whether it is a simple cleaning, the
filling of a cavity, or a surgical procedure. Your doctor or dentist will prescribe an antibiotic to reduce
the risk of endocarditis, which is an infection of the
heart's inner lining or valves. Your dentist can give
you information about dental hygiene and check
dentures for proper fit, especially if you are having
difficulty in chewing.
- **Look for an aphasia support group.** You may consider participating in an aphasic program conducted
by a speech and language pathologist in your local
hospital or other facility.

Getting the Most from an Office Visit

An office visit should give you a chance to ask all the
questions you may have. Perhaps some subjects were previously discussed but need to be repeated outside of the
hospital setting. It is an opportunity for you and your
family to learn more about your condition, ongoing care,
your medications and side effects, and any difficulties you
are experiencing. It is also a time to talk about your concerns, and to set realistic, personal goals.

The average office visit with a doctor lasts about eleven
minutes, so it's a good idea to figure out beforehand what
you want to accomplish. Here are some strategies to consider:

- **Go to the doctor with a family member or friend who makes you feel at ease.** This helps you stay relaxed and focused, which can help you get what you want out of the visit. Write down questions, or keep them in your mind, and put the important ones first. (Suggested questions to ask the doctor are on pages 149–152.) Your companion can write down the answers the doctor gives to your questions and can help remind you of things you wanted to discuss.
- **Try to keep records to chart your progress, and discuss them with your doctor.** Your doctor may recommend that you keep a record of your medications and side effects, your blood pressure, diet, physical therapy, and exercise. It also may be extremely worthwhile for you, a family member, or other assistant, to keep a record of changes in your condition—including any pain you're experiencing—so that you and your doctor will be able to note problems and progress.
- **If your doctor uses medical jargon that you don't understand, ask for an explanation.** If you don't understand, don't be embarrassed to ask!
- **You are entitled to copies of your medical records.** If you need to consult another doctor for a second opinion, or if you need to change doctors, it can save time and money already to have the information that is needed.
- **Take some food to tide you over.** Be prepared for the possibility of a long wait. Bring snacks—nutritious ones, of course. Also, be sure to bring any medicine you may need to take during this time.

TAKING CHARGE OF YOUR MEDICATIONS

Stroke may happen suddenly, with no prior warning. However, for more than 2.5 million Americans who have survived one or more strokes, there usually were years of a slow buildup of fatty deposits inside the blood vessels. This condition is called atherosclerosis.

More than half of all people treated with stroke take as many as three or more medications, some for a combination of concurrent medical conditions. According to the Framingham Heart Study, the first large-scale study designed to determine the causes of atherosclerotic heart disease, stroke rarely occurs in isolation: 67 percent of all stroke survivors have high blood pressure, 47 percent have coronary heart disease, and 32 percent have diabetes.

The medications prescribed for the combination of conditions often found in people who have had a stroke need to be taken two or three times a day—some with food to avoid stomach upset, others before meals on an empty stomach. To further complicate what is already confusing, several pills may look exactly alike. It's not easy to remember to take the right medicine at the right time and in the right amount for the right length of time prescribed, particularly when someone has a memory deficit!

Almost 2 billion prescriptions are written in this country each year, and 50 percent do not produce the desired results, either because incomplete instructions are given or because the instructions are forgotten or not fully understood. The label may not include complete information concerning the name of the drug and how it should be taken, such as with or without food and in relation to other drugs. Many over-the-counter products—particularly aspirin and products containing aspirin (such as Alka-Seltzer, Midol, cough medicines, and allergy products)—can increase the anticoagulating potential of anticoagulants and cause excessive bleeding. Ibuprofen and indomethacin (sold as Nuprin, Advil, Indocin, Motrin, and other brands) also interact with anticoagulants. Some foods, vitamins, and alcoholic beverages can interact with certain drugs and cause troublesome side effects. Also, some drugs need to be refrigerated, whereas others are kept at room temperature.

To help keep track of medications, the Rusk Institute recommends these general guidelines:

- **Plan to take medications at the same time each day.** It's a good idea to get into the habit of taking your medications at the same time each day when you do some other routine task, such as at mealtimes, either before or after eating.
- **Try to take your medications on time.** It's important to take medication at the right intervals, but a half hour early or late usually isn't crucial. If you are more than several hours late in taking a medication, ask your doctor if you should omit the dosage altogether or double it the next time.
- **Keep a chart to manage your medications.** A handy way to keep track of all the medications you take is to keep a chart. A sample chart you may want to use as a guide is on the following page. List the medications you are taking, the time they are to be taken, and check each dosage off as you take it. If you skip a dose, for whatever reason, place an "X" in the appropriate box to indicate a missed dose. Write down any side effects, or ask a family member or other assistant to keep a record so that you can report them to your doctor.
- **Bring your medication chart with you to discuss it with your doctor.** If you are having difficulty with a medication, call your doctor immediately rather than waiting until your next appointment.

- **Color-code your medicine containers.** If you have trouble reading the labels, you may want to color-code the containers or identify them by touch. For example, wrap a rubber band around one medicine bottle, and glue a piece of emery board to the top of another. Make a note on your medication chart of the code that you use.

- **Use a seven-day pill organizer.** Plastic containers with compartments divided and marked for morning, noon, night, and bedtime can be purchased in most pharmacies and health-food stores. They're also available by mail from Bruce Medical Supply (800-225-8446) for less than $10.

- **Try an electronic pillbox which beeps as a gentle reminder.** Set for any schedule, an electronic pillbox gently signals you when to take your medications. It shows the day and time you last opened the box and even flashes to indicate if you missed a dose. Electronic pillboxes are available at Radio Shack; other brands may be obtained from your druggist or through mail-order companies. An alternative and similarly helpful idea is to wear a wristwatch with an alarm to remind you to take your medicine.

- **Keep a backup supply of medicine wherever you spend time away from home.** Not only is it convenient, but it can also be extremely important to keep a small supply of medicine anywhere you regularly spend time away from home. For example, if nitroglycerin is prescribed, carry several tablets with you at all times, and keep a backup supply at any place besides home where you spend time. Nitroglycerin is effective for only about 3 months and must be replaced regularly. Warm weather can affect it, so it may be helpful to date the container in which you keep the nitroglycerin tablets, or any other medications that are not viable beyond a certain date.

159

A CHART FOR RECORDING YOUR MEDICATIONS

Month Of: _____

MEDICINE	Day		1	2	3	4	5	6	7	8	9	10	11	12	13	14	15	16	17	18	19	20	21	22	23	24	25	26	27	28	29	30	31
		AMT																															

Morning / Afternoon / Evening

Instructions: Write in your medicine and the amount you are to take. Put in the day of the week in the box under the date. Place a check in the appropriate box after taking the medicine. Place an **X** in the box to indicate a missed scheduled dose.

Selecting a Pharmacy

Surveys show that when a prescription is to be filled, most families take it to the pharmacy closest to the doctor's office or to the one closest to where the person lives or works. Thus, convenience is one of the things to consider when choosing a pharmacist. Here are some other factors involved in selecting a pharmacy:

- Are the prescriptions competitively priced? Does the pharmacy offer discounts?
- Can the pharmacist be reached easily by phone? When an emergency occurs during the night, on a weekend, or during a holiday when the store is closed, what provisions are made to make medicine available? Do they deliver? How long does it take for a delivery, and on which days or nights are deliveries not made?
- Does the pharmacist keep a record of all your prescription medicines, your nonprescription medicines, and any allergies you may have to certain medications? (Some states require that records be kept so that the pharmacist can give advice about medication uses and possible interactions. But in reality, you are still responsible for having this information about each of your own prescribed medicines.)
- Does the pharmacist offer to answer questions and give you instructions about the prescribed medicines?
- Will they accept your prescription insurance plan?
- Can you use a credit card to charge your purchase? Can you be billed monthly and pay by check?

You may decide to buy your medications in larger quantities from a discount house or order through the mail, especially if a prescription is expensive, needs to be reordered repeatedly over a long period of time, or if it is not fully covered by insurance. See page 227 for information about the mail-order pharmacy service of the American Association of Retired Persons, (202) 434-2277.

READING ABOUT YOUR MEDICATIONS

To supplement what you learn from your doctor and pharmacist, ask if there is any written information about your specific medications that you can take home with you. The pharmacy may also have available at the counter various reference books or computerized drug information.

Pharmacists use the *United States Pharmacopoeia,* which is generally considered one of the most influential resources for standards and information on prescribed drugs. It has monthly updates. One volume is specifically for consumers and provides comprehensive data about a medication, its purpose, how to take it, frequent and even rare side effects, and interactions with other medications. It is usually available to be read by consumers at the counter.

PHONING YOUR DOCTOR

When you arrive home from the hospital, the primary communication link with your doctor is the telephone. In the past, you probably called your doctor infrequently. Now you and your family may find the need to call more often.

Ask your doctor about the best time to call for non-emergency matters. Some doctors set aside early-morning hours to receive calls. When you leave a message, ask when you can expect to hear back from the doctor. Your call should be answered within a reasonable length of time. If necessary, call again to make sure your message was received.

Here are some tips to get the optimum quality from your telephone communications with your doctor:

- Write down the questions you want answered and keep them in front of you. You'll feel calmer and more organized with your thoughts on paper.
- Keep telephone conversations as brief as possible, but make sure they are long enough to accomplish the purpose of your call.
- When you call the doctor's office, you may speak to a nurse who can give you answers to some of your questions and will refer others to the doctor.
- When a prescription is needed, give the doctor the phone number of your pharmacy or ask your pharmacist to call the doctor. If the prescription cannot be filled over the phone, arrange to have someone pick up the prescription from the doctor's office, deliver it to the pharmacist, wait for it to be filled, and then bring it to you.
- To be prepared for an emergency, write down the following information and keep it close to the phone so it can always be easily located. Use large block letters so that you can read it even without your glasses.

1. **your doctor's phone number**
2. **the 911 number or the number for Emergency Medical Service in your community**
3. **the hospital emergency number**

4. **the telephone numbers of people whom you want notified in case of an emergency. (For more about handling an emergency, see chapter 3, "Being Safe," page 79.)**

EVALUATING YOUR RELATIONSHIP WITH YOUR DOCTOR

While you were in the hospital, you were cared for by many doctors. Now that you're at home, your relationship is with one or two doctors, usually your family physician or internist and a neurologist. Since you may spend considerable time on the phone and in the office with these doctors, your personal relationship with them is important. For this reason, it's a good idea to give some thought to how you are getting along with your doctors. Talk the matter over with your family and friends. You cannot succeed optimally in your healing process unless you have confidence in the relationship. Here are some questions you may want to consider for yourself:

- Do I have confidence in the doctor?
- Do I believe the doctor is caring?
- Would I recommend the doctor? If yes, why? If not, why?
- Does the doctor listen attentively and fully grasp what I say?
- Does the doctor encourage me to ask questions? Do I understand the answers?
- Does the doctor give me enough time or do I feel rushed?
- Am I encouraged to be fully involved in my care? Am I given all the information I need?
- Does the doctor encourage me to get a second opinion when a medical procedure or surgery is recommended or if I am in conflict about my treatment?

Margaret Lewis*, Whose Husband Had a Stroke

My husband is now sixty-four, and he had a stroke two months ago. Our biggest problem is that it's very difficult for him to speak. He was a seller and designer of fabrics; he was the vice president of a major firm. His bread and butter was communications. He ran a sales force of many, many men. He went around the country speaking and presenting things, in addition to designing textiles. So this speech disability was devastating.

We're using a local rehab center where they come with a van to pick him up. When I go to see his therapists there, I feel absolutely a part of his therapy work. You see, I'm very assertive with this. I was there for the first week and a half watching everything and telling the therapists what I wanted.

> "My goal is to get [my husband] to the best that he can be, and I don't care who I have to fight to get it..."

My goal is to get him to the best that he can be, and I don't care who I have to fight to get it—I don't care that they have the degrees. And I'm going to get it. So I have to be on top of his rehab care at all times. In physical therapy, they had him walking around. I don't need them walking him around because he already walks around. I'm using them for the best that I can get out of them as professionals to bring him back to where he should be. They hadn't been giving him the bike, and he wasn't getting much exercise. I told the physical therapist that I would like to have him on the bike. "Well, that's okay, too,

* This is a pseudonym.

but we want to have him doing other things," was the reply. I said okay and waited about a week, but I didn't see any progress with the other things. There was a little stretching, a little walking. But I looked at the bike and I said if he was able to walk with the muscles he used on the bike, I wanted him to have some time on the bike. And finally—by pushing—I got it.

You think that because they're trained they're always doing the right thing. Well, my father and uncle were doctors. What I heard years ago was, "Well, when the doctor makes a mistake, he buries it." That stayed in my head. So I like a recommendation from somebody I respect. Then when I get names I look them up in my medical directory. Who are they, where they got their training, their qualifications for the type of thing they're going to be doing. I look them up. I also have a *PDR* [*Physicians Desk Reference*]. Doctors are only human, and so are the therapists.

When you get home, you have to stay on top of the therapy. You have to educate yourself or you may only get second best.

Chapter Six

Lifelong Learning

You can learn to follow the inner self... Healing is simply attempting to do more of those things that bring joy and fewer of those things that bring pain.

—O. CARL SIMONTON, M.D.

No Two People Are Alike

We each have our own plan for living in the world, even if it isn't articulated—and we draw upon whatever strengths we need to get us through. An inner clock produces our own personal time schedule, particularly during recovery. No matter what the statistics indicate, physical and emotional healing takes place in its own time. We're entitled to heal at our own pace.

Recovery and adjustment for a person who has endured a stroke is dependent on many factors: the specific site and severity of the brain injury; the person's general health, personality, and determination; the support of family and friends; and the quality of medical care and rehabilitation.

"In this country, you're allowed a short period of time to grieve, and then you're supposed to pull yourself up by your bootstraps and get on with it," says Rosalie Longoria, who had a stroke at forty and is also diabetic. "It takes a long time to really believe that you can have control of your life even with a disability. And when you realize you can direct your life—even if you don't do everything on your own—you begin to have a life again."

What does it take to bring about positive changes in your life? How do you reestablish a balance when you feel depleted by physical and psychic wounds? How do you take charge of your life after stroke? Who are the people who can help?

"A stroke scares you so much. It makes you take a look at your life, perhaps as never before," says Michael Ajamian. "You begin to realize fully that your life is yours and not your family's or your doctor's, even though their support makes a big difference. But you're the only one who can decide how you will live your life. I had the same feelings as someone who faces a terminal illness. For me,

the losses were the use of my right hand, and some language and memory impairment," Ajamian continues. "I
felt everything very intensely—shock, denial, rage, and
depression."

Natalie DiMico, whose stroke followed a heart valve
replacement when she was sixty-two, believes that "it's all
prayer. Let's face it, this isn't something you do alone.
Rehabilitation continues forever; and you bring the same
willingness to do a good job with it as you have brought
already to whatever else you have accomplished in your
life."

PRIORITIES ARE PERSONAL

With his two sons about to enter college, Michael Ajamian's first priority was to get back to work. "It was at the
top of my list; whoever could help me do that was someone I needed." Ajamian was overcome by a series of set-
backs, among them depression, tremendous fatigue, and
a lack of stamina. It took about a year before he could
return to running the family business of supplying equipment for bakeries.

For six months, there were physical, occupational, and
speech therapy sessions three days a week at a local rehabilitation center. Transportation provided by the center
relieved his wife, Nina, from having to make the trip and
wait until he finished, usually in the late morning. At
home afterward, Ajamian would prepare his own lunch
and take a much-needed rest.

During the early period of his recovery, he spent a good
deal of time with his brother-in-law, who had recently
undergone cancer surgery. "Walking and talking with
Tim, we sorted out the problems of the world, ours in-

cluded," Ajamian says. "We decided we loved life even
when we felt sick and depressed."

For Arthur Marantz, however, the focus has been on
relearning a wide variety of skills in order to be independent in his daily life. With weakness on his left side, physical, occupational, and speech therapies began almost at
once in the hospital. Three weeks at a rehabilitation center in his community increased his confidence.

For Marantz, his physical therapist has been a strong
influence. "His therapist is the sister of his former secre-
tary," says Bryna Marantz, his wife of thirty years, "and
knows him well enough to tap into what motivates him.
The physical and occupational therapies gave him back
his ability to manage his own life within the limitations of
his injury."

Bryna finds that "life since the stroke feels as though
I've been handed a script I hadn't studied. Looking at
Arthur, you never would suspect he had a stroke. He has
no paralysis, he is outgoing and generally in good spirits.
Yet we have traded places in our traditional roles."

The responsibilities for their personal investments and
managing their home and other property are hers for the
first time in their relationship. "When we go out to dinner,
I do the ordering and pay the check—which sometimes
causes some surprised glances! He finds it too confusing
to read the menu, handle money, or sign a credit card,"
Bryna says.

"Until my doctor read the riot act to me and explained I
was placing my physical and psychological health on the
line, I was a part of almost all of Arthur's waking hours.
Gradually I've been scheduling companions to take my
place so I have some time off. Some are friends, others are
paid helpers, and this has meant a period of adjustment
for us both."

Once it's no longer a life-and-death situation, Bill Ryan,
a psychologist, says the first questions asked of therapists

by virtually everybody are: "How long is this going to last?
How permanent is it? Am I going to show improvement?
If so, how much and how long will it take? What can I do
to help?"

Dr. Ryan continues: "These are very complex and emotionally charged questions, and we spend a lot of time
with the person who has had a stroke and their family
trying to explain and support each one until they get a
firm handle on it. Once we get beyond that, we discuss the
functions which are likely to change, versus those that
may take longer."

POSSIBLE CONSEQUENCES OF LEFT-BRAIN AND RIGHT-BRAIN INJURY

Although symptoms of brain injury vary widely depending upon the part and severity of the injury, some general-
izations can be made. A common way of characterizing
stroke injury is by the particular side of the brain that is
affected. A stroke will not affect all areas of the brain.

An injury to the left side of the brain that results in
paralysis—temporary or always—will affect the right
side of the body. A right-sided paralysis is the result of
injury to the left side of the brain. Certain definitive types
of language problems and changes in behavior are also
associated with left-brain or right-brain injury.

Most people with left-brain injury have some degree of
aphasia, or difficulty in speaking and/or comprehending,
and it will manifest itself differently in each person. The
complexity of the problems reflect the intricacy of the
communication process. It involves creating and organizing a thought, finding the words to express it, and pro-
ducing the words; it also involves perceiving that

someone wants to say something to you, following the words as they are spoken, and then understanding the meaning of the message.

The most dramatic changes occur in the first three to six months of recovery; smaller changes may continue for long afterward. Most of today's poststroke rehabilitation supports the notion that if one area of the brain is damaged, other centers can assume the role of the injured tissue. One purpose of therapy is to both bring out the potential of these uninvolved centers and provide the stimulation to permit the brain to reorganize and adapt.

Here are some of the symptoms of left-brain and right-brain injury that people who have had strokes may experience.

Left-Side Brain Injury

Paralysis or weakness on the right side of the body.

Right visual field cut or deficit.

A portion of the area on the right side of the person's vision is blank, and the person is unaware of the change. Objects on the left side can be seen more easily. There may also be tunnel vision, blurring, and double vision.

Speaking and listening.

People with right hemiplegia are likely to have problems with speaking and understanding. Their ability to understand may be greater than their ability to speak. (This consequence is slightly less certain for those who are left-handed.)

They may have trouble pronouncing words.

There may be a problem with the continuous repetition of particular words or phrases.

They may have memory problems related to language and recalling names and nouns.

They may have difficulty in naming objects, although their use may be understood.

Reading, writing, arithmetic.

There may be problems with reading and writing. Some may communicate better by writing; with others, spoken communication works best.

There may be problems with writing or gesturing (express aphasia) and/or difficulty in understanding written or spoken language (receptive aphasia).

Activities of daily living.

There may be right-side neglect (although this is less severe and long lasting than left-side neglect in right-brain injury).

Some people have trouble performing tasks such as dressing and those related to personal care.

Emotions.

Some people experience feelings of despair and hopelessness, and so they may cry easily or become easily angered.

Slow, cautious, anxious behavior may be noted.

Right-Side Brain Injury

Left-sided weakness or paralysis.

Arm, leg, and frequently both are affected.

Left visual field cut or deficit.

A portion of the area on the left side of the person's vision is blank, and the person is unaware of the change. Objects on the right side can be seen more easily. There may also be tunnel vision, blurring, and double vision.

Awareness of the left side.

The person may neglect or ignore the left side of the body and environment.

They may comb their hair, shave, and apply makeup only on the right side.

They may eat only the food found on the right side of the plate.

They may read and write only on the right side of the page.

They may bump into furniture or other objects on the left side.

They may have difficulty steering a wheelchair.

Faces may be hard for them to recognize.

They may experience disturbances in the sensation for pain, as well as hot and cold, on the left side.

Speaking, reading, writing, arithmetic.

The person's speech may be imprecise—slurred and difficult to understand.

They may be unusually talkative, repeating the same words or phrases over and over again.

Their speech may lack inflection, cadence, and appropriate melody.

There may be problems with reading and following the lines of a paragraph.

They may read without understanding the meaning of what was read.

Listening and conversation.

Their impaired listening ability may make give-and-take in conversation difficult.

Their conversation may be self-centered.

They may have a tendency to continue talking without giving another person a chance to talk.

Eating and swallowing.

They may have chewing and swallowing difficulties.

Orientation, visual perception, judgment.

The person may have problems judging depth, distance, and direction.

They may have difficulty in recognizing or perceiving familiar forms, objects, and information; in some instances, they may have difficulty recognizing familiar faces or discriminating among people in general.

They may be unable to use money, make change, write checks, or dial a phone.

They may have a tendency to become lost when outside of their own immediate environment.

They may be able to follow instructions only if they are given in simple, single steps, with time to complete one step before the next is attempted.

They may have difficulty dressing, putting on clothing in the wrong order and not recognizing the error.

They may be unable to recognize time on a watch or clock.

They may have problems with the concepts of time and space.

They may experience a loss of musical abilities.

Attention and awareness.

The person may have a short attention span. (For some, this problem may be extreme.)

They may not be aware of their own errors or may act euphoric when it's inappropriate.

They may have problems completing a task.

They may be unable to discern relationships and associations.

They may have trouble synthesizing, abstracting, or organizing information.

They may appear to be intent on performing a task but may not, in fact, follow through.

There may be lack of awareness of personal limitations, accompanied by a denial of problems.

They may claim to be engaging in activities like driving or shopping when they aren't, in fact, doing so.

They may be unable to do activities that require full and focused attention.

Emotions.

The person may laugh inappropriately.

They may exhibit abrupt, impulsive behavior.

They may talk too much or too little.

They may be emotionally flat or have difficulty showing emotions.

They may be unable to discern easily the emotional content in other people's voices. Expressions, emotions, and nuances in facial gestures such as a raised eyebrow may go unnoticed or unperceived.

They may have problems with uncontrolled swearing or bursts of angry words.

They may make inappropriate and untimely yet all-too-true disclosures.

EMOTIONAL REACTIONS AFTER STROKE

"Perhaps one of the most bewildering changes for someone recovering after a stroke, and for his or her family, is
the rapid, exaggerated, and inappropriate mood swings
experienced by their loved one, often accompanied by
outbursts of tears, laughter, or extreme anger," notes Dr.
Ted Rule, a neuropsychologist. He explains reflex crying
by using the example of when the doctor hits your knee
with a reflex hammer, causing it to give a little jerk. The
spinal cord carries out this reflex; the brain is not involved. The highest level of the brain, the cortex, inhibits
or dampens reflexes that are controlled by the spinal cord
and the lower parts of the brain or brain stem. When the
cortex of the brain is damaged, these reflexes—no longer
inhibited—are released.

"Your leg jerks when the hammer hits your knee, even
though you don't give your leg the command to kick," says
Rule. "In the same way, the crying reflex is triggered even
when you don't have the full set of emotions that might
usually go with it. Just as the knee-jerk reflex requires the
stimulus of the hammer and doesn't occur randomly, so
too does the crying reflex require some stimulus to be
triggered. Reflex crying needn't be as intensely felt as
something that would customarily bring about tears. Still,
there is some emotion connected to it."

Dr. Rule believes that the crying is often neither a reflex
nor tied to extreme feeling but is a blend of both. Over
time, episodes of inappropriate crying, laughter, and anger diminish, as do unaccustomed feelings of suspicion
and overwhelming sadness.

"It takes a long time to know what you need," Tom
Watson asserts. "At first, being so sick means you are
never able to keep up with your own needs. Maybe you
shouldn't even try to put your needs into words. In time
you discover them—if you give yourself the time and
space to make the discovery."

Says Watson, "I am certain of one feeling: loneliness. It makes you doubt who you are and what your life is worth. So how you go through that dark tunnel and come out the other end, how you feel about what has happened to you, and who urges you on make all the difference. There's no telling who it will be who gives you the will to go forward. It could be your wife or husband, children, grandchildren, friends of many years, God, or people you meet with experiences similar to yours. What has been most important to me is to know that the people dear to me think of me as having a future—which I've earned."

Here are some recommendations for family and friends on dealing with the emotional reactions of stroke:

Ask the person what would comfort them.

At a time when the person isn't crying, ask them how they would like you to handle it when they cry. Some people prefer that you not call attention to them when they're crying; they would rather have you distract them with conversation because they find their crying stops more quickly when they are diverted. Other people may want you to help them in different ways.

Empathy and understanding are always welcome.

Whether the tears are a reaction to some particular upset or are reflexive, acknowledge them by saying something like "I can see how difficult things are for you right now and how hard you are trying." A good gauge of what is appropriate is any genuine expression you would like to hear if the roles were reversed.

Be respectful of the feelings.

Because of their own discomfort at seeing their loved one crying, family members may be tempted to look away, or leave the person alone. Unless the person has specifically stated that this is what they prefer, stay nearby, remain calm, and be as supportive as possible.

Crying has restorative powers.

Researchers have discovered that crying has both a psychological and physical healing value. It is an important way to release tensions and relieve emotional stress.

You can learn more about brain-behavior relationships from professionals.

The primary-care physician, neurologist, neuropsychologist, and occupational therapist can give you specific information about emotional distress, anxiety, and inflexible or rigid thinking and can also recommend strategies for coping with them. Even if you've never before considered psychological counseling, it may contribute significantly to the quality of life for everyone in the family.

Getting Up When You're Feeling Down

Few men and women who survive a stroke escape a sense of emotional upheaval. It varies only in its intensity and the length of time it lasts. Emotions are often conflicting and confusing. Feelings of sadness, guilt, impatience, helplessness, loss, depression, love, and dislike may coincide with one another. You may tell yourself some of these feelings are "good" and others are "bad."

Many stroke and aphasia club members say that regardless of how you label them, all the feelings experienced are valid and a natural reaction to what you've endured. "Feelings are there, and it's best to put your effort into coping with them, instead of judging yourself for having them," says Rosalie Longoria.

"Some families may not recognize depression as a real problem and may tell their loved one to 'snap out of it,' place blame, or believe that the person could be happier if they only wanted to," Longoria says. "Depression, however, is very painful and needs to be treated as no less serious than any physical problem."

She suggests giving your doctor every opportunity to help you directly, since he or she may be able to tell you about how others in similar situations to yours have managed or may refer you to specialists who can help. If your doctor doesn't respond in ways that are comforting to you, go further. You may want to see a neuropsychologist experienced in working with people who have had a stroke.

Other stroke club members represent another option for comfort and support. They can provide reassurance that your emotional reactions are shared by many. In listening to others, you can actually hear yourself, but with a new perspective.

Find support.

Put yourself in situations where your abilities are validated. Try to be around people who make you feel good about yourself. Turn to friends for advice about reaching your goals; then consider their recommendations and decide what you think is best for you.

The best medicine is often a good listener.

Research shows that people who can express strong feelings of grief and anger, resentments, and fears survive adversity better than those who are emotionally constricted. It may help to have a close friend or confidante with whom you can share every day. Some stroke clubs have outreach programs, while some community organizations, churches, and synagogues have volunteer telephone reassurance programs.

Celebrate your victories.

Every gain is hard-won. Pause to celebrate your accomplishments. Watch out for professionals who use self-limiting words and labels. Progress will come, even if it comes slowly. Always take note of how far you've advanced.

Insist on being a contributing member of the family.
Don't let anyone take away your role in the family and
the responsibilities that you can handle.

Be determined.
Survivors intuitively operate on the persistence
principle—it's always too soon to quit. Fierce determination helps overcome many kinds of adversity and produces results.

Believe you can make a difference.
Researchers studying the characteristics of optimistic
people find that they believe in themselves having both
the will and the way to accomplish their goals, whatever
they may be. Even when up against considerable difficulties, they tell themselves that things will improve with
time, and they will have played a significant role in that
progress.

Helping someone else also helps you.
Healing often comes through an awareness of others.
Making a commitment to another person can counter the
inclination to become resigned and bitter.

Judge whether you can control a situation.
If you feel you have some control over a situation, there
is less likelihood of becoming depressed. You are more
likely to move into an action mode—rather than dwell on
a problem—if you believe you can influence the outcome.
No matter how challenging life becomes, decisions or
choices always can be made.

Acknowledge the tough times.
When you and your family undergo times of stress, it's
important to take time out to share the feelings in order to
see how they can be resolved. Bottling them up can just
lead to frayed nerves and misunderstandings.

Anger can be harnessed.
Anger, although often experienced as a raw and painful
emotion, can also be used as fuel to ignite the determination to survive. Look for signs of anger such as impa-

tience, uncooperativeness, sarcasm, hyperawareness, and bitterness and turn its power to your advantage.

Make peace with your mistakes.

To reduce your feelings of depression, you need to learn to tolerate your mistakes without being unkind to yourself. You don't have to like making mistakes, but you can accept them when they happen and treat yourself fairly when they do.

Most of our stress comes from what we tell ourselves.

Often, what we say to ourselves is not empowering, not constructive, and is a source of stress. Learning to speak respectfully to yourself—being a friend to yourself—is one way to counteract the negative interior dialogue. For most people who are experiencing depression, mornings are the hardest times. With the whole day's tasks ahead, it is a good time to substitute affirmative thinking for negative "self-talk."

Break up large tasks into more manageable basic components.

It is easier to harness your power for problem-solving if you are not overwhelmed by the contemplation of one large goal. Instead, take it one small step at a time.

Consider professional counseling.

Even if you've never before considered psychological counseling, you may want to see a therapist who is experienced in working with people who have experienced a medical crisis—especially specialists in stroke.

Look for professionals with whom you can be honest.

Look for medical professionals you have confidence in and with whom you feel comfortable enough to be candid. You know when it is that you find people whom you can work with successfully and who have your best interests at heart.

Establish relationships with other people who have had strokes.
Listening and sharing within the community of stroke clubs and aphasic groups can provide enormous strength and support. When you are ready, reach out to help someone else who may still be struggling with some of the obstacles you've already overcome.

Ask yourself how you can gain from this experience.
We all like to be able to understand why something "bad" happened. But it is possible to make the transition from defeat to power by shifting the focus from why it happened to what you can do to triumph over it.

A WELLNESS PROGRAM

A number of stroke risk factors are the same as those for heart disease, although their relative importance varies. Research supports the view that coronary artery disease can be controlled and reversed. Because three of the greatest risk factors for stroke—high blood pressure, heart disease, and diabetes—often do not cause symptoms in their earliest stages, it is essential that someone who has had a stroke have regular screenings for these and other cardiovascular risk factors.

Lifestyle choices that contribute to the risk of stroke include smoking, excessive alcohol consumption, and the use of cocaine and amphetamines. Oral contraceptives, personality type, geographic location (especially the southeast, sometimes called "the stroke belt"), certain types of climate, seasons, and even socioeconomic factors are thought to contribute to the relative risk of stroke. Also of some significance are age, gender, race, familial, and genetic factors.

About 1 percent of people between ages sixty-five and seventy-four have a stroke, and 5 to 8 percent of people in that age group who have had a ministroke go on to stroke. Although the risk associated with advancing age cannot be reversed, the awareness of it figures importantly in planning preventive therapies.

Reducing Risks and Setting Personal Goals

Stop smoking. Men studied in the Framingham cardiovascular disease research project who smoked more than forty cigarettes a day had twice the stroke risk of men who smoked fewer than ten. In a Harvard Medical School study of women, the number of cigarettes smoked was found to be directly related to stroke risk. Women smoking more than twenty-five cigarettes a day had 2.7 times greater risk of stroke from a clot or embolus, and a 9.8 times greater risk of a hemorrhagic stroke. Five years after stopping, ex-smokers have a stroke risk equal to that of nonsmokers.

Eliminate the excessive intake of alcoholic beverages. Drinking in excess does considerable damage to all the body's systems, including the vascular system—the one most significantly involved in the incidence of stroke.

Try to reduce total serum cholesterol to under 200 mg/dl with a total cholesterol/HDL ratio of approximately 3.5 or less. Research indicates a link between high blood lipid levels and atherosclerosis in cerebral arteries, but it is still unclear whether high cholesterol levels significantly increase stroke risk. They do, however, increase the risk of heart disease, so efforts should be made to reduce them.

Achieve a normal blood pressure of 140/90 or better. Even mild elevations in blood pressure are associated with an increased risk of stroke. High blood pressure is present in 50 to 70 percent of stroke cases, depending primarily on the type of stroke. Sometimes mildly elevated blood pressure can be controlled by lifestyle modifications, but medication is often needed. Blood pressure can be raised by a person's being inactive, overweight, and ingesting salt in excess amounts. Lower blood pressure levels are associated with a marked decrease in the occurrence of stroke.

Exercise and maintaining ideal weight reduce many health risks. Obesity and physical inactivity are risk factors for stroke primarily because together they increase the risk of high blood pressure, heart disease, and diabetes. They also may be independent stroke risk factors. Maintaining body weight within 5 percent of the normal range reduces the risk of high blood pressure, high blood cholesterol, and type II diabetes and provides cardiovascular improvement.

Reduce the risk of heart disease. Strokes are a strong risk factor for heart disease, and heart disease, in turn, increases the risk of a stroke. People with coronary heart disease, congestive heart failure, enlargement of the left side of the heart, disease of the heart valves, or irregular heart rhythms have a several-fold increase in the risk of stroke.

Heart disease is associated with stroke in two ways. First, damage to the heart such as from a heart attack may make it more likely that clots will form within the heart. These clots can break loose and travel to the brain, causing a cardioembolic stroke. Also, heart disease and stroke are linked because they are both evidence of atherosclerotic disease in the blood vessels. If the blood vessels feeding the heart—the coronary arteries—are diseased, it is likely that arteries to the brain are also affected.

Maintain blood sugar levels. People with diabetes are at risk for stroke, just as they are for heart disease. Women with diabetes are at even greater risk than men. High blood pressure compounds that risk. Control of high blood sugar—hyperglycemia—can reduce the severity of cerebral damage during a stroke.

Learn techniques to reduce stress levels. Complement good-quality medical care with relaxation breathing, meditation, visualization, biofeedback, psychological counseling, mutual help support groups, and prayer. They can calm the mind and soothe the spirit.

WHAT'S LEFT TO EAT?
STRATEGIES FOR TURNING GOOD INTENTIONS INTO HEALTHY EATING

There is a natural tendency in most people after a stroke to want to make radical lifestyle changes, especially in their diet. Actually, the fewer radical changes you make, the better your chances are for adhering to a new diet. Start by looking at what you're doing right. It may take less of a major overhaul to achieve your goals than you imagined.

By now, almost everyone knows the golden rules of healthful, defensive eating and weight loss: use less fat in cooking and at the table. Choose fresh fruits and vegetables over processed foods. Switch from high-fat whole-milk dairy foods to low-fat and nonfat milk, cheese, and yogurt. Eat less meat, and try more fish and dried beans for sources of protein. Check the labels of salad dressings, canned soups and gravies, crackers, bread, cookies, and cakes for their salt and fat content—and for the types of sweeteners, additives, and preservatives they contain.

So why aren't we all eating wisely? Partly because knowing what is best for us and actually doing it are two different matters. Change is hard-won, even when we know the food we eat can harm us.

Millions of men and women who have had a stroke and

who also have high blood pressure, a heart condition, and/or diabetes have decided that their lives depend on what food they eat and have worked out a plan they can live with. This doesn't happen by itself, and it's never easy. They begin by substituting more wholesome foods for ones that are off-limits. Family recipes are translated into healthier versions. The butter and shortening once used for frying become oil sprayed or wiped lightly across a nonstick pan. Fruit juice, low-sodium tomato and vegetable juices, sodium-reduced soy sauce, and wine replace the fat used for sautéing. No longer sabotaged by cholesterol-free claims alone, informed consumers pass up unhealthy products by scrutinizing labels for the presence of unwanted hydrogenated vegetable oil, palm kernel oil, and coconut oil.

Men and women recovering from a stroke who are also coping with other medical conditions discover that in order to have variety and flavor without the added fat, salt, and sweeteners found in commercial products, their food needs to be prepared the old-fashioned way—that is, "from scratch." Start to look at the products you usually buy without changing everything at once. Most people are willing to give up a certain food if another is offered in its place. Consider your options in buying food similar to your traditional fare without the hidden sources of fat, salt, and sugar. You might decide to make your own salad dressings, quick soups, and desserts so that you don't have to give up eating all the foods you enjoy.

Reading the Labels

Labels seem deliberately baffling. Some say that this is so because the food industry would lose billions of dollars if consumers knew the real amount of fat, salt, sugar, additives, and preservatives contained in the food they serve their families.

Information on the label is divided into two categories. The first is the nutritional information for each serving. This includes the number of servings in the container, the serving size, the calories in each serving, and the protein, carbohydrate, and fat content of each serving in grams. The second category states the percentage of the U.S. Recommended Daily Allowances (U.S. RDA) which the product provides. Label ingredients are listed in order of decreasing weight—the first ingredient present has the highest weight, and so on.

If any nutritional information is on the label, the amounts of vitamins A and D, thiamine, riboflavin, and niacin must be listed as a percentage of the recommended daily allowance. Two minerals, calcium and iron, also must be listed. Protein must be shown as a percentage of the U.S. RDA, as well as in weight by grams. As many as twelve additional vitamins and minerals may be listed if the manufacturer chooses to include this information. Fresh meats, poultry, fish, fruits, and vegetables are usually not labeled, but packaged foods—cold cereals, canned goods, and so on—are.

Fats. Dietary fats, as well as oils—which are a form of fat—can be classified as saturated, polyunsaturated, or monounsaturated. Most fat-containing foods, even those such as oils, which are 100 percent fat, contain a mixture of these three. Some of the words on food labels which indicate that fat is an ingredient include safflower, coconut, corn, and olive oils, lard, butter, shortening, margarine, suet, lecithin, egg yolks, lipid, tallow, monoglycerides, diglycerides, triglycerides, polyunsaturated oil, and hydrogenated or partially hydrogenated vegetable shortening.

Calculating the fat content of food: Most food labels list the calories in a serving and the grams of carbohydrates, fat, and protein. To calculate the percentage of calories in the serving provided by fat, you first convert the weight of fat in grams to calories of fat. The conversion factor is 9, meaning that 1 gram of fat contains 9 calories. In other words, 5 grams of fat in a serving would equal 45 calories.

If the total calories per serving is 120 and the fat per serving is 8, then 8 grams of fat per serving times 9 calories per gram equals 72 calories of fat. This means that 72 of the 120 calories are fat calories. To find the overall percentage of fat, divide 72 calories by 120 total calories, which equals .60, or 60 percent.

If you want to know the percentage of fat quickly, without having to do the arithmetic yourself, you can buy a nonelectronic calculator called the Percent-O-Fat Calculator, available in health food stores for $5.95. (If you can't find it in your health food store, call the manufacturer, APR Industries, at 1-800-266-3733.)

The two general classes of fat: Animal fat is solid at room temperature and is highly saturated. The most familiar fat from animal sources is found in red meat, poultry, butter, cheese, egg yolks, lard, and whole milk.

Vegetable fat is liquid at room temperature and includes both polyunsaturated and monounsaturated fats. Polyunsaturated fats are liquid at room temperature and even at cold temperatures; they include soybean, sunflower, cottonseed, and corn oils, as well as the oils found in almonds, filberts, and pecans. Monounsaturated fats are also liquid at room temperature, although they may become solid in the refrigerator. Major sources of these are derived from avocado, canola oil, cashews, olives, olive oil, peanuts, peanut oil, and peanut butter. Both polyunsaturated and monounsaturated fats contain the same number of calories as saturated fat—9 calories per gram—and are 100 to 125 calories per tablespoon.

Hydrogenated vegetable shortening is a solid fat created by adding hydrogen to a vegetable oil. Margarine

would be liquid without hydrogenation. Most hydrogenated fats are not tallied up separately on the nutrition
labels. The words *hydrogenated, partially hydrogenated,* or
hardened are used to describe oils on the ingredient label.

There are also some naturally occurring highly saturated vegetable fats. These include coconut, coconut oil,
cocoa butter, and palm oil. These fats contain no cholesterol, but evidence has shown that they do raise blood-
cholesterol levels.

Salt. The "code names" for salt on labels include sodium chloride, sea salt, kelp, baking powder, baking soda,
monosodium glutamate (MSG), sodium saccharin, sodium nitrate, sodium propionate.

Sweeteners. Sweeteners have words ending in *-ose,*
such as sucrose, lactose, glucose, and fructose. Other
names for sugar and sweeteners include corn or grape
sugar, corn or grape sweetener, corn syrup, cane sugar,
brown sugar, raw sugar, sorghum, molasses, honey, sor-
bitol, and mannitol.

AEROBICS: THE EXERCISE OF CHOICE

The majority of people who have had a stroke choose to
take regular walks around the neighborhood or inside a
nearby shopping mall early in the morning before the
stores become crowded. Still others choose to rebound in
a well-supervised exercise program, a senior exercise program, or a supervised program at a local Y.

Aerobics is the exercise of choice for cardiac fitness.
Walking, water aerobics, swimming, and low-impact aerobics are all aerobic exercises that start to burn fat at an

early stage of the training session and ensure a constant supply of oxygen to the muscles.

Aerobics literally means "with oxygen." To qualify as aerobics, an activity—if performed regularly—must be rhythmic, involve the arms and legs, and be maintained for an extended period of time in order to increase the body's cardiovascular endurance.

The Foundation of an Exercise Program—"FIT"

In addition to the type of exercise that you do, three basic variables must be considered when you develop an exercise program based on the information you have been given by your doctor. The variables can be expressed in the following way: *frequency* (how often you work out); *intensity* (how strenuously you work out); and *time* (how long you work out). One way to remember these variables easily is by thinking of them as the acronym FIT.

Frequency. How often you exercise is one factor in generating good results from an exercise program. Generally, exercise should be done at least four times weekly or, at most, six times weekly, with at least one day of rest.

Instead of waiting until you next see your doctor to begin your exercise program at home, call with any questions you might have about the workout you are planning to do.

Intensity. Intensity is determined by your target heart rate and the data calculated from your response to the treadmill exercise test. For most people, this is the highest rate achieved during the test; for others, it is the highest heart rate that occurred in the absence of angina or abnormal blood pressure response.

Intensity is expressed in terms of the maximum heart

rate, which is determined by subtracting your age from 220. The maximum heart rate for a 60-year-old, for example, would be 160. Working out at a target heart rate of between 60 percent and 75 percent of the maximum rate—which is the recommended intensity for nonathletes by the American Heart Association—the pulse range would be between 96 (160 × .60) and 120 (160 × .75) beats a minute (which is the pulse), respectively. Your doctor will advise you of the range in which you should work out. Undoubtedly you will build on this as you become more fit.

An expenditure of 2,000 calories a week through exercise is generally considered sufficient. You expend about two calories a minute walking two miles an hour. At three miles an hour, the expenditure is about five calories a minute.

As your fitness level improves, you will need to increase the intensity to maintain your target heart rate. As you notice this change, consult your doctor about the improvement and ask for instructions about increasing the intensity of your exercise.

Time. Depending on your stage of recovery and whether or not you have had cardiovascular surgery, your level of fitness will determine how long you will be able to exercise. It can range from 15 or 20 minutes for beginners, up to 45 minutes or longer as you build your endurance.

The time refers to the actual time that you are within the training heart-rate zone, and does not include a warm-up or cool-down period.

Warm-up Period

A warm-up consists of walking at a pace of about 7 to 10 minutes below the training heart rate (that is, about halfway between your resting and training heart rates).

In cold weather, increase the length of your warm-up by five minutes to ensure that there is an adequate blood supply to your heart and working muscles. If you have hypertension or if you experience cramping in your legs, take 7 to 10 minutes in warm weather and add an additional 5 minutes in cold weather.

Warming up starts channeling blood to working muscles and causes the heart and respiration rates to start a gradual rise; it also helps stiff muscles and joints to limber up. To prevent injury, it is advisable always to warm up your muscles before stretching them. Stretching may also be done at the end of the exercise session, immediately after your cool-down period.

Aerobic Exercise Program

The most beneficial portion of the exercise program for developing the heart and circulatory system is the exercise session itself. Since your workouts must be continuous, your training heart rate provides a safe means to monitor yourself.

Check your individual exercise prescription for your training heart rate and the specific duration of your workout. To gauge if you are working hard enough to accomplish your fitness goals and yet not too hard to be unsafe, take the "talk test." If you are working out at a reasonable rate of aerobic exertion, you will be able to talk—although you will notice an increased rate of breathing and some perspiration. If you have difficulty talking, pull back until you reach a safe aerobic exertion rate for yourself.

If you have been inactive for a long time, have arthritis or another orthopedic condition, are extremely overweight, or if you have given up exercise because of exhaustion, pain, or to avoid possible injury, begin by gradually incorporating additional activity into what you do every day. For instance, start by parking your car a few blocks farther away than you normally would; take the stairs instead of the elevator; or walk at a purposeful pace for 5 to 10 minutes.

Cool-Down Period

Just as the warm-up period is gradual, your cool-down period allows the heart rate and blood pressure to return to their resting states. Stopping suddenly will cause blood to pool in your legs and may make you feel light-headed. In hot or humid weather, increase the length of your cool-down to assist your body in returning to its resting levels. Take your pulse to check your recovery heart rate after 5 minutes. If your heart rate is still above one hundred beats per minute, continue to walk slowly until it slows down.

Wait at least 10 minutes to shower or bathe after exercise in order to allow all your body functions to return to a resting state. Keep the water at about body temperature, not excessively hot or cold. Water that is too hot slows the circulation and can cause dizziness, and cold water can strain your heart.

Taking Your Pulse

You can count your own heartbeat by taking your pulse. The number of times you feel the pulse in a minute is your pulse rate. Your pulse rate is the same as your heart rate. When you take your pulse, you can feel your artery give a little jump each time your heart beats.

Some people take their pulse before getting out of bed every day, before taking certain medications, and before, during, and after the cool-down stage of an exercise session. Ask your doctor when to count your pulse and whether you should keep a record of your pulse rate.

- Using the pads (not fingertips) of your first two fingers, find your pulse at either the carotid artery (at the neck) or the radial artery (at the wrist).
- Press lightly until you find your pulse, especially at the carotid pulse, since pressure on this artery can sometimes slow the heart.
- Begin counting when the second hand of a clock or watch is at a point where a 10-second interval will be easily distinguished.
- Starting with the number 0 as a baseline, begin counting the number of heartbeats felt for a 10-second interval. Multiply this number by 6 to get your pulse rate for one minute.
- Take your pulse before, during, and after exercise to monitor your exercise properly.

If you have difficulty taking your pulse and you want to make sure you are maintaining your target heart rate, consider buying a watch that takes a reading of your pulse. Casio makes a watch that indicates both blood pressure and pulse. Sporting equipment stores usually stock it as well as other brands of this item. The watch is also available by mail order from Self Care at 1-800-345-3371 for $149.

Exercising is of greatest value when your heart rate stays within your safe "target zone"—high enough to stretch your capacity but not too high to be of concern. You can program your target zone into a heart-rate monitor that you wear on a comfortable chest belt—worn over a T-shirt—that beeps a sound if you go beyond it. Electronic sensors accurately measure your actual heartbeat and you see the results on an easy-to-read wireless wrist display. Sporting-goods stores usually carry heart-rate monitors. Or call Self Care at 1-800-345-3371 to order a Polar Heart Monitor for $169.

Exercise and Weather Conditions

When the weather is hot, you should exercise during the cooler times of the day, such as in the early morning or late evening. Potential heat stress will occur in high temperatures, high humidity, and low wind, so exercise outdoors in a hot climate only if you are very fit and used to the heat.

During the cold months, dress in layers so that clothing can be removed or added as needed. Choose light clothes that "breathe." Make the first layer of clothing a material that wicks away moisture from the skin, such as polypropylene. Wool makes an excellent second layer. Keep layers loose in order to trap your body heat and act as insulation. The first thin layer removes perspiration from the skin, the second provides warmth, and the third protects against wind and rain. Some people like a pair or two of cotton or wool socks. Others prefer a thin liner made of polypropylene undersocks made of wool or synthetics. Wear a cap or hood and mittens (mittens are warmer than gloves) made of wool or synthetics to prevent excessive loss of body heat.

If you develop angina in cold weather, check with your doctor about exercising outdoors. You can protect yourself from cold air by wearing a ski mask or a scarf pulled loosely in front of your face when you are active in the cold. Breathing warm air will often reduce or prevent anginal attacks.

If the day is windy, the first segment of the exercise session should be taken into the wind. That way, on the return trip, excessive fatigue and chilling due to walking or running into the wind can be avoided.

Going the Distance

Begin gradually and attempt to build exercise into your regular schedule. Choose the kind of activities you enjoy, and stay with it even if at first you don't see marked results.

Choose the time of day that suits you best. If you exercise as soon as you get up in the morning, you have the advantage of being rested. If you exercise before you shower and dress for the day, it saves you the energy and effort of showering and changing clothes later on.

The exercise prescription given you by your doctor is uniquely yours. Based on your level of fitness, your medical condition, and the results of exercise tolerance tests, your prescription will tell you how often, how hard, and for how long you will need to exercise.

Stay within your prescribed limits. Train regularly without excessive peaks of activity. Avoid intensive competition. Never be out of breath or unable to carry on a conversation.

Learn your training heart rate. By knowing the desired level of intensity of your workout and by checking your pulse, you have a safe and effective means of monitoring your efforts. If you check your pulse, and it is above your target heart rate, simply slow down.

When you have a minor illness accompanied by a fever, do not exercise. After a minor illness, resume your exercise program cautiously. If you miss more than a week of exercise, cut your program back by one-third when you begin again. You lose fitness about twice as fast as it takes to build it up, so don't be concerned if it seems to be taking a long time to get back into shape after you've been out for a while.

Wear a Medic Alert identification. Also, carry money with you for a phone call or to take a bus or taxi ride home if you become overtired.

Know the signs and symptoms that must be reported *immediately* to your doctor. Here are some of them:

angina (chest pain)

light-headedness or dizziness

feelings of nausea or vomiting

leg cramps (claudication)

breathlessness lasting more than 10 minutes

confusion or disorientation

palpitations

loss of color in the face or bluish skin tone

abnormally high blood pressure

Delayed symptoms that last at least a day should also be reported to your doctor, including:

excessive fatigue that lasts a day or more and that continues even after you have slept well

difficulty in falling and staying asleep

persistent racing heartbeat

fluid retention accompanied by weight gain

Ask your doctor for safe exercise guidelines. Ask how long you should wait after eating before doing any strenuous exercise. Discuss the number of times you should work out each week and the appropriate intensity level at which to exercise. Establish how long each exercise session should last.

Air pollution causes difficulty in breathing. In extremely hot or cold and windy weather and when there is smog or other excessive pollution, walk indoors in a mall, at home on a treadmill, or ride a stationary bike.

Drink plenty of water. To avoid dehydration, drink a glass of water 15 to 20 minutes before you exercise, even if you are not thirsty, and drink small amounts of water—4 to 6 ounces—at 10-to-15-minute intervals during the exercise session, especially if you are perspiring. Dehydration can cause an elevation of your heart rate. Continue to drink water after the completion of your exercise period.

Setting Personal Goals

In setting your goals, make them specific and measurable. Keep them realistic by using guidelines from your doctor and physical therapist. For example, you might want to set as a goal your desire to take a walk 4 or 5 times a week; another may be to set aside a specific time each day to carry it out. If one of your goals is to lose weight, you may want to ask your doctor or a nutritionist if this can be attained in the time you have set for yourself. Use the same guidelines for other goals you have in mind.
Your Personal Goals:

_____
_____
_____

Enlist the support of family and friends. Enthusiasm is contagious, and it's pleasant to have someone along. It also keeps you on track to have an exercise partner.
List the people who can join you in exercising.

_____
_____
_____

Keep track of your progress. Write down or ask someone to make a note of how you respond to the workout, particularly if you experience pain or excessive fatigue, and discuss this with your doctor. Make copies of the weekly exercise plan on page 00 or design your own chart if you prefer.

There is a weekly exercise plan on the following page. If you make copies and fill it in, you can keep track of the amount of exercise you are getting and your progress. You may want to take your chart with you when you see your doctor to discuss your exercise plan.

Suspend all self-criticism. Make the time you exercise a gift that you give yourself. Feel pride in your accomplishments, and trust yourself that you are giving your body what it needs in order to repair itself.

Focus on one goal at a time. It is more effective to concentrate on a single goal than to diffuse your energies.

Reinforce successful experience. Figure out what you can achieve, and gradually upgrade your efforts at planned intervals.

COUNTDOWN TO STOP SMOKING

In his book *The No-Nag, No Guilt, Do-It-Your-Own Way Guide to Quitting Smoking,* Dr. Tom Ferguson says that most nonsmokers simply do not know how best to help a health-concerned smoker. He suggests that "hard sell" approaches, which produce guilt and shame, can be counterproductive.

The following guidelines are for family and friends who wish to lend support to smoker's efforts to reduce their health risks and are adapted from Dr. Ferguson's book:

Separate the smoker from the smoking. Let your relative or friend know that you will continue to care about them no matter what they decide to do about their smoking.

202

Week of: **EXERCISE PLAN**

MONDAY	TUESDAY
YOUR COMMENTS:	
PULSE: During Exercise After Cool-Down	PULSE: During Exercise After Cool-Down

WEDNESDAY	THURSDAY
PULSE: During Exercise After Cool-Down	PULSE: During Exercise After Cool-Down

FRIDAY	SATURDAY
PULSE: During Exercise After Cool-Down	PULSE: During Exercise After Cool-Down

SUNDAY	Target Heart Rate: _____
	Range: ____ _____
	Personal Goals:_____
PULSE: During Exercise After Cool-Down	

Try to see the problem from the smoker's point of view. If you attempt to look at how the person feels about smoking, it may help you to have a better understanding and increase your tolerance. Smoking may be such a cherished part of someone's lifestyle that to give it up would feel like losing a good friend.

The temptation simply to ignore the negative health effects of smoking can be very strong. The physical and psychological addiction can be so powerful that quitting can be painfully difficult. Smokers who do not have the courage to confront this dilemma deserve compassion and understanding, not ridicule and blame. A supportive relationship with a caring and understanding nonsmoking friend can make the smoker feel more secure and, at the same time, provide the positive psychological motivation for change.

Encourage the smoker to do what they think is best. It is only when someone really wants to do something about smoking that progress can occur. Instead of telling smokers what to do, encourage them to do what *they* think is best.

Suggest sports and other enjoyable activities not conducive to smoking. Since sports are incompatible with smoking, as are activities such as concerts and religious services where smoking is not allowed, they may stimulate the smoker's motivation to stop.

You have rights as a nonsmoker. You can ask your relatives and friends not to smoke in your presence or in your house or car, but you should do so in a polite, nonjudgmental way.

What follows is a "Countdown to Stop Smoking" chart. You may want to make copies of it, and wrap it around a pack of cigarettes.

COUNTDOWN TO STOP SMOKING

Week of: _____

	Write in Time	Place	Situation and Feelings	Rating 1–4	Alternatives to Smoking
MON.					
TUES.					
WED.					
THURS.					
FRI.					
SAT.					
SUN.					

Instructions: Make a photocopy of this chart and wrap it around your pack of cigarettes, holding it with a rubber band. If you unwrap the pack and smoke a cigarette, or take one offered by someone else, complete the information. Note the time, place, situation, and your feelings. Give each cigarette you smoke a rating: 1 is a cigarette you feel you can't do without; 2 is less necessary; 3 is a cigarette you could really do without; 4 is a cigarette you are not really sure about. This chart helps you to understand why and when you smoke and to create alternatives to smoking.

RETURNING TO WORK

Considering Your Options

"Will it be possible for me to return to work?" is one of the primary questions most people who worked before their stroke ask their doctor. Typically, if being employed is viable, the doctor's answer will be based on your condition, how far advanced you are in your recovery, and the kind of work you do.

Generally, people do not go into great detail with their doctor about their jobs. The whole area of work and its stresses can go unnoticed, especially if the doctor adheres strictly to answering medical questions. Most doctors are hesitant to introduce these personal subjects, fearing that doing so would invade a person's privacy, as well as being outside of their usual realm. You or a family member may need to initiate a discussion with your doctor about your concerns, if you are considering returning to work.

You may not have considered talking to your doctor in this way because of physical disabilities or communication problems, or because you feel unable to do the same work as before; or you may be hesitant because of other less well formulated concerns. Transportation may be a seemingly insurmountable obstacle, and work disincentives may make working financially impractical. You may be unfamiliar with the American Disabilities Act, which protects the civil rights of citizens with disabilities and extends its protection into the workplace.

Rosalie Longoria, a magazine editor who returned to work one year after her stroke, says she still accomplishes a great deal but now works differently than before. Longoria works out of her home on a computer linked to the office; a fax machine and overnight mail delivery are the other two indispensables in making her new work situation possible.

Hank Mills, a vocational rehabilitation counselor, believes that some men and women who worked before their stroke could return to the work force but hesitate because they may not know how to approach the challenges as well as the services and accommodations available.

Supported employment, for example, is a program offered by a number of nonprofit organizations such as the Head Injury Association and Independent Living Centers. They offer one-on-one coaching, retraining of skills, and assistance in securing and maintaining employment.

Occupational therapists in rehabilitation settings and in private-practice work with individuals to see what their needs are in the workplace. They guide them in finding easier ways of working and in gradually building stamina. In some instances insurance will cover the training costs if it leads to a return to full employment.

"You may want to talk to a job coach or vocational rehabilitation counselor to learn about job-training opportunities in your area, and to learn about your rights as a disabled person," Mills suggests. If your job is in jeopardy because of your disability, talking to a professional will help you to make informed choices and put you in touch with advocacy services that may be useful.

Mills recommends that when considering continuing your present work or changing to something different, you should list your physical capabilities and limitations. Factor in your energy and endurance, your communications skills, and how you feel these will impact on the way you handle your work. Realistically evaluate your type of work, any work disincentives, the day-to-day stress factors, and the relative accessibility of transportation.

If you apply for disability benefits, you are considered eligible for services provided by your state's vocational rehabilitation agency whether your claims are approved or not. These agencies offer counseling programs and guidance, job training and placement. In some states, however, a financial means test is required for vocational training, support services, and job placement. There are also private career counseling services available, and it is best to choose one that has experience working with employees with disabilities.

To learn about your Social Security benefits, you can call the Social Security Nationwide Toll-Free Telephone Service at 1-800-SSA-1213 or 1-800-772-1213. You may be entitled to supplemental security income or disability benefits. This agency can send you free literature on retirement benefits, disability benefits, Medicare, and survivor benefits.

For information about your employment rights, transportation accessibility, and accommodations to support you at work, call your local Independent Living Center (for more about these centers, see page 218) and the Job Accommodation Network (JAN).

The Job Accommodation Network—JAN—funded by the President's Committee of Employment of Persons with Disabilities, has human factor consultants who will refer you to appropriate agencies for job-training programs and information about employment opportunities. The organization does no job placement. Instead, its main function is as an information resource on the American Disabilities Act and the laws that protect citizens with disabilities. JAN may be reached at 918 Chestnut Ridge Road, Suite 1, Morgantown, WV 26506, (800) 526-7234, and can send you its catalogue of books, pamphlets, and audiovisuals, as well as a copy of the American Disabilities Act.

Looking at Work

Here are some things to consider when contemplating your possible work options:

- Can I do the work I once did? Is it possible for me to return to the same job?

- Can I work part-time? Can I work at home?
- Should I do another, less demanding kind of work than what I did before, even if I am paid less?
- What kind of retraining do I need now in order to do my work?
- What are my financial resources? Do I have enough to cover my needs on a long-term basis if I am unable to have the same earning power?
- What am I entitled to get in unemployment insurance and disability benefits? Am I entitled to any supplemental Social Security income?
- What are my work disincentives? Will working cause me to lose my disability benefits?
- How do I want to spend my time? Do I want to spend my time differently than I did up to now? What are the interests that I'd like to pursue?
- How are the other people in my family or whom I live with affected by the changes in my work life?

Tips from People Who Have Had Strokes, Who Are Employees and Volunteers

Be flexible. Think of new ways to make changes in the way you work. (Can you work shorter hours, less intensely, and so on?)

Pace yourself. Take time out to rest. Stick to regular, consistent hours, without extending them to overtime.

Take your medicines on time, especially if you're busy. Keep a backup supply of medications at work. Make taking care of yourself a priority.

Communicate what you need at work. If you have a tendency to take on everything and do it all yourself, get some assistance. For example, if there are any helpful adaptations or devices that could make your job easier and help you work more efficiently, discuss them with your employer.

Some people will treat you differently when you return to work because of their own insecurities about illness. Make every effort to be a part of the activities at work. Expressing your interest in people you work with promotes a sense of belonging. Use humor or a light attitude when dealing with a person who seems newly uncomfortable in your presence. If you feel the relationship is valuable, try to confront the person and talk it out.

Take short breaks. Take time to rest and renew yourself. Learn some relaxation techniques. Try these: Breathe gently, then exhale slowly through your mouth. Pay attention only to your breathing and block everything else out. Get up and move to another place in the room (even if it's only in your imagination). Talk to yourself in a positive, encouraging way. (See page 252 for books and audiotapes on meditation and other stress-reducing techniques.)

Consider professional psychological or vocational counseling. It may put into perspective some of your concerns about work. Appropriate support groups may also offer tools to cope with work-related problems.

If you are continually upset by your supervisor, notice how the person deals with others. You may not be their only target, and perceiving that will help you take the assaults less personally. Think of ways to improve the situation for yourself.

Trust your judgment about setting your own limits. You are the only one who knows what works best for you.

Have a life after work. If your work is especially stressful, plan noncompetitive leisure sports and relaxing activities in your time off from work.

INTIMACY AFTER A STROKE

"The odds against you keeping your relationship going the way you want to are so great, that when you're successful, you feel a little smug!" says Michael Ajamian. He recommends asserting your right to retain your role in the relationship with your spouse—even if your roles are seemingly reversed.

"Keep your self-esteem intact by being independent, even if you are being assisted with many things. And watch out for the parent-child roles which are easy to fall into when a mate assumes caregiving responsibilities, because with it you could relinquish your sexual role."

Ajamian continues, "A time for intimacy needs to be scheduled—sexual spontaneity mostly happens in the movies! Arrange for a private time together to rest, relax, resolve your conflicts, and be intimate. Recall a particularly special time in your lives together and try to recreate it. Go back to a favorite restaurant or listen to some music you both enjoyed. Set aside a few minutes each day to say something nice to each other. Don't go to bed angry with each other. Do whatever it takes to bring you closer to each other, and to take the focus off illness."

"Your partner is just as scared as you are," says Barbara Faye Waxman, a disability consultant in sexuality, reproductive health, and family life rights. "You are entitled to go at your own pace, but you need to let your partner know what that pace is. Resuming your sexual life is a very essential part of healing," Waxman continues. "Receiving love and giving love and expressing your sexuality play a very large role in feeling fully alive again. Test the waters first. The first thing you may want to do is just touch and cuddle, and that may continue for a while. Intercourse may be something for later on."

If you have feelings of anxiety about resuming your sexual life, you are not alone. After a stroke, men and women alike worry if it will ever again be safe for them to engage in sexual activity. In his book, *Heart Illness and Intimacy: How Caring Relationships Aid Recovery*, Dr. Wayne Sotile—a psychologist and family and marriage therapist—answers some of the questions and concerns people have about the safety of sexual activity. "Although the sexual response cycle results in cardiovascular changes, the changes are not different from those experienced during regular exercise. The average heart rate during lovemaking is 117 beats per minute, while blood pressure increases to a maximum of $145/87$ during a typical sexual encounter."

"Start by asking your doctor for information and assurance," Barbara Waxman suggests, "and then go further for the support which you can get from people who have had a stroke, and are working through the same issues. Local stroke clubs and coronary clubs are excellent sources for personal information."

The basic concerns of men and women differ only slightly. While a man may be troubled for varying periods of time by impotency and premature ejaculation, he may also have to adjust to more passive positions in order to place less strain on his affected side or on a painful shoulder and to conserve his energy. Before the stroke, these positions might have been unacceptable, but they are now necessary to achieve intimacy and sexual satisfaction with his partner.

A woman who has had a stroke may react for a time with general sexual dysfunction—particularly in terms of being aroused and in reaching orgasm. Problems in communication, concern about attractiveness, loss of sensation, or the presence of a catheter can contribute to altered desire.

After a stroke, many people find that there is so much else to deal with that sexual feelings are "walled off." Sexual drive, attributed in part to hormonal changes, is affected after stroke. Some medications suppress the sexual drive along with pain and other sensation, or cause communication problems, anxiety, and other difficulties. Similarly, chronic depression—prevalent after a stroke—

can contribute to disharmony in a relationship. Sexual problems may be reflective of only one aspect of an inability to experience pleasure.

If no one introduces the subject of intimacy in an office visit, or if a doctor hesitates to ask probing questions for fear that a discussion of sexuality will be perceived as an invasion of privacy, the problems will remain and can do more damage over time if left unresolved.

Dr. Wayne Sotile recommends that if you and your partner have questions and concerns about sexual intimacy that would take longer to answer than the time allotted for your usual visit, ask your doctor for another appointment for the specific purpose of discussing this matter. Prepare for the appointment by composing a list with your partner of what you would like to discuss. Talking with your doctor can probably be reassuring and helpful. If you or your partner feel uncomfortable at the idea of talking with the doctor, you might want to consider seeing a marriage and sexuality therapist or a neuropsychologist.

DR. JEROME WEISNER, PRESIDENT EMERITUS OF THE MASSACHUSETTS INSTITUTE OF TECHNOLOGY

I think every stroke is different. And I think there are a lot of things people don't know about the brain and strokes. My brain was able to react and make it possible for me to do things that I couldn't do at first.

> "...I was never discouraged because people were always so patient with me."

When I woke up from the stroke, I wasn't able to speak or walk or use my left hand. I had a very, very good therapist who worked on my speech and my spelling, and I find that after nearly three years, I'm still learning, improving. For example, I couldn't spell anything—even two-letter words. In fact, I had to learn the alphabet all over. But I was never discouraged because people were always so patient with me. Many people, of course, don't have that sort of speech problem with a stroke; it depends on where the stroke is. It took me many months to learn to spell two- and three-letter words with the help of an unusually good therapist. I learned to use my arm again using a lot of technology, but I still can't use the fingers of this arm. I'm still working on it. I have the feeling from my own experience that some parts of the body adapt more readily than others. And also I think it's a matter of luck. For example, when people told me to do things even when I couldn't talk about them, I knew what they were telling me to do.

When there's an assault to the brain, other parts may compensate by adaptation. It takes training and practice to stimulate and enhance those adaptive abilities. For example, I don't think I've worked as hard on my fingers as I have on my speech. And I think it shows. In other words, if I had put the emphasis on using my left hand and fingers instead of learning to speak and write, I think they would have been better. For me, it was much more important to learn to communicate again than to use the left hand. But now I can't use my hands for anything, because it turns out that one hand is not enough to do most of the things I want to do. Now I'm starting to spend more time on it. I've been writing, oh, maybe an hour a day, on the computer for two reasons. It allows me to use only one hand, and it's easier; also, my spelling is not as good as I would like it to be either, right now. The computer has a spelling corrector. So when I can't manage a word, I can easily find it.

I still get very tired since my stroke. I've talked to a specialist about this and he said that anybody who's had a brain injury uses a lot more energy than a person who hasn't had a stroke. Before I had my stroke—I had my stroke when I was seventy-three—I used to be able to go around the world, and stay up until two or three in the morning, and still function. The first couple of years, I found myself not only fatigued but very anxious when I had to talk. But just two days ago, I went to a meeting which I was very interested in, and I found that I had much less of the anxiety when I had to talk. In fact, I didn't have any of the kind of anxiety that I had always had when I tried to talk before. So as far as I can tell, things are still improving.

Chapter Seven

Information, Services, and Products

Experience is not what happens to you; it is what you do with what happens to you.
—ALDOUS HUXLEY

Family members, friends, neighbors, and coworkers will often ask, "What can I do to help you?" Much of the material in the preceding chapters is for you, the person who has had a stroke, or for the person who lives with you. But this chapter provides an opportunity for others to help without much inconvenience to them, since in many cases the calls can be made from home or office. Perhaps it would be a good idea for a family member to be in charge of coordinating this "research team." And as with all work of this type, everyone feels gratified by participating in such a worthwhile project.

FINDING COMMUNITY RESOURCES

When you need outside help but you aren't sure where to go for it, or even what to ask for, a local organization that provides information and refers you to the appropriate agency is your best bet.

- **The telephone book is a good starting place.** Most phone books have a section of blue pages listing area agencies. In the Yellow Pages, look under "Social and Human Services." Many communities and organizations also publish a telephone directory listing community support services exclusively. Looking at the listings of organizations helps to begin the networking process that is usually necessary to find what you want.
- **Chapters of the American Heart Association have information about stroke.** Organizations that serve a medical condition make referrals to community organizations, services, support groups, resources,

and counseling for individuals and families. The
American Heart Association has pamphlets on
stroke, aphasia, diet, high blood pressure, brain-
behavior relationship, and sexuality which they can
send you on request. For the **American Heart Association's Stroke Connection**, call (800) 553-6321,
Monday through Friday, 8:30 A.M. to 5:00 P.M., central time, for information about stroke groups in
your community.

- **An Area Agency on Aging is an excellent resource
  for local organizations.** The Agency funds a variety
  of community services for the elderly. More about
  their services may be found later in this chapter under
  "Support for Caregiving Families" on page 224.
- **Many home health-care services are available in
  every state.** Public agencies, private organizations,
  and volunteer groups all provide services. There is no
  central agency that coordinates or evaluates all
  home-care services.

  The hospital discharge planner, your doctor, family, and friends are good sources for recommendations of home-care agencies. If nursing and physical
  therapy have been prescribed by your doctor and you
  know that these services will be covered by your insurance, you must use only those agencies approved
  by your insurance in order to be reimbursed.
- **Independent Living Centers are an excellent resource.** There are two hundred nonresidential centers across the country run by disabled consumers
  who coordinate or directly provide services such as
  transportation, job counseling, psychological support services to families, and peer support, as well as
  a list of experienced personal care aides. To find a
  nearby Independent Living Center, call or write to
  Southern Tier Independence Center, 107 Chenango
  Street, Binghamton, NY 13901, (607) 724-2111.

- **The Health Information Center, (800) 336-4797, locates health information through the appropriate national organizations, associations, clearinghouses, and self-help support groups.** The Center is a program of the Office of Disease Prevention and Health Promotion, P.O. Box 1133, Washington, DC 20013.
- **Local Mental Health Associations are a good referral source.** The associations will make referrals to their member therapists. For more about mental-health resources, see page 223. See also the Associations for Physical and Occupational Therapy and Social Workers on page 221.

HOME-CARE SERVICES

Nursing

If nursing services have been ordered by your doctor, or you and your family would like to hire a nurse, many options are available.

The private duty Nursing Registry at the hospital will arrange for a nurse to accompany you home. Your local Nursing Bureau of Nursing Registry, whose address and phone number can be found in the Yellow Pages, will send a nurse to your home upon a simple phone request.

Visiting Nurse Associations and other nonprofit groups will usually send a nurse for a single, approximately one-hour visit, but the for-profit, private home-care agencies will also arrange for shift work, if it is requested, just like the service that is provided in the hospital.

Shift work is usually done in eight-hour blocks—7 A.M. to 3 P.M., 3 P.M. to 11 P.M., and 11 P.M. to 7 A.M. Especially during postoperative care, several home visits can give the family the necessary confidence to manage. The nurses can evaluate and assess the care that is needed and teach any required procedures. If the nursing services are reimbursable by insurance, the home-care or nursing agency must be from an approved agency. For more about home-care services, see page 130.

Personal-Care Aides

In any community, several sources exist for finding personal-care assistance. By calling a full-service home-care agency, you should be able to obtain a personal-care aide. The agencies interview and train the aide, and a nurse supervises in your home from time to time.

Most home-care and nursing agencies will not send a personal-care aide for less than four hours a day. If you want to interview the person beforehand, you may be charged the four-hour minimum, so ask about this.

Many families decide to recruit, train, and manage a personal-care aide *outside* of the auspices of an agency, although it may take considerable time to locate a person who is reliable, trustworthy, and pleasant. Often a family member, friends, or neighbors know of someone they can recommend. Or another good place to ask is at a stroke meeting. Many people also get helpers and other assistance from nonprofit organizations, such as the Independent Living Centers.

• **ADAPT (American Disabled for Attendant Programs Today), 12 Broadway, Denver, CO 80203, (303) 733-9324**, is a consumer advocacy group that has information about personal-care aides and your rights as a home-care client.

VISUAL REHABILITATION

"An uninformed person may say to someone who has double vision after a stroke, 'Learn to live with it' or 'close one eye to see better,' " asserts Dr. Harold Friedman, Chief of Visual Therapy Service at the State University of New York School of Optometry. "It's very possible to deal with double vision on a much more constructive level with appropriate prisms and lenses, and sometimes with visual exercises, if the condition is not too severe."

Eye-care professionals who specialize in visual rehabilitation and offer options for people with the common visual changes of stroke can be found in every state. There are seventeen schools of optometry all over the country, and they can refer people to professionals who work with prism lenses. "But you must contact the correct person since not every school of optometry has visual rehabilitation staff members. Another source is an association of optometrists in your state," Dr. Friedman advises.

ORGANIZATIONS AND ASSOCIATIONS

• **The American Physical Therapy Association, 1111 North Fairfax Street, Alexandria, VA 22314, (800) 999-2782 and (703) 684-2782.** Registered physical therapists and assistants are licensed and regulated by the states. The Association is a good source of information about physical therapy and will refer you to your state association. Most states require that you be referred by a doctor. The departments of physical therapy in hospitals and rehabilitation centers are good referral sources, as are members of stroke and aphasia clubs.

• **The American Occupational Therapy Association, Inc., P.O. Box 1725, Rockville, MD 20849-1725, (301) 948-9626.** This professional association has information and printed materials about occupational therapy. Occupational therapists may require that you be referred by your doctor. The occupational therapy departments of hospitals and rehabilitation centers are good referral sources; so are members of stroke and aphasia clubs who can recommend therapists they themselves have worked with.

• **National Speech-Language-Hearing Association, 10801 Rockville Pike, Rockville, MD 20852, (800) 638-8255, and (301) 897-8682** (both are voice/TDD), is a national organization that provides information and answers questions about all speech, language and hearing disorders. The organization provides professional referrals throughout the country.

Nutritionists and Registered Dietitians

Almost anyone can call himself or herself a nutritionist since licensing is not required. Most legitimate nutritionists are likely to be members of the Society of Nutritional Education, the American Institute of Nutrition, or the American Association of Clinical Nutrition, which have strict entry requirements.

• **American Dietetic Association, 216 West Jackson Boulevard, Suite 800, Chicago, IL 60606. Their consumer hotline is (800) 366-1655 or (312) 899-0040.** They will send you the names of registered dietitians available for consultation in your area, if you send them your request plus a stamped, self-addressed business-size envelope.

Psychological Counseling

Your doctor and therapists are a good source for a referral to a neuropsychologist or clinical social worker experienced in working with stroke survivors and their families. Your local Mental Health Association can also make referrals for practitioners in your area, as well as for support groups. Your state's psychology licensing board, which may be listed in your telephone book under state government agencies, is another source of referrals.

Finally, hospitals, medical centers, and the rehabilitation institutions affiliated with academic medical schools are referral sources. Most hospitals have therapists on their staff who provide individual and family therapy, as well as stress-reduction programs, biofeedback, relaxation techniques, and peer counseling. Most home healthcare agencies and Visiting Nurse Associations have social workers on staff.

• **American Association of Sex Educators, Counselors and Therapists, 435 North Michigan Avenue, Suite 1717, Chicago, IL 60611, (312) 644-0828.** This association will make referrals to its members, who are counselors experienced in sexuality problems related to physical illness.

• **Local chapters of The American Psychiatric Association can give referrals.**

• **National Association of Social Workers (NASW), 750 First Street NE, Washington, DC 20002, (800) 638-8799.** NASW, which is the largest professional association of professional social workers, will direct you to your state chapter. Clinical social workers work in hospital settings and in private practice.

SUPPORT FOR CAREGIVING FAMILIES

It is estimated that as many as ten million people between ages forty-five and sixty care for a dependent relative or older adult. Recent studies show that about 65 percent of all American caregivers are under sixty-five; over 40 percent hold full-time jobs.

• **The hospital social work department can provide you with information and refer you to community services.** While you are in the hospital, you can get a wealth of free information from the social work department. With your permission, the hospital discharge planner will arrange for home-care services.

• **Local libraries have useful resources.** Here you are likely to find the names, addresses, and telephone numbers of community organizations, as well as a listing of the services available in your area. The National Library Service for the Blind and Physically Handicapped, Library of Congress, provides braille and recorded books and magazines, catalogs, music scores, and music instruction material free for blind and physically handicapped persons. Talking-book players and accessories, necessary to use the cassettes and records, are also provided without cost.

• **Your doctor, his or her nurse, or assistants may recommend organizations and services.** You may get good leads on services that others have used and recommended to the staff.

• **The Area Agency on Aging (AAA) sets up needed nonmedical services.** This organization is a governmental agency that funds community home-delivered meals, free transportation to doctors' offices, shopping and housekeeping help, and social activities, among other functions. They can refer families to companies that manage and provide professional home-care services, including nurses, personal-care aides, and physiotherapists. Some AAAs provide financial-planning assistance or will advise you where to find it. You can find the agency listed in the Yellow Pages of the telephone directory under "Social Service Organizations" or a "Guide to Human Services."

• **Community Ys have many programs.** In addition to classes, workshops, and low-cost sports programs for families, many Ys have programs for senior citizens that combine social and educational activities, as well as exercise.

• **The National Rehabilitation Information Center (NARIC), 8455 Colesville Road, Suite 935, Silver Spring, MD 20910-3319.** NARIC is a national rehabilitation library and information center that collects and disseminates data from commercially published books, journal articles, and audiovisuals. The collection covers all aspects of rehabilitation and disability, including independent living, employment, medical rehabilitation, and legislation.

• **ABLEDATA** can be reached by calling NARIC at (800) 346-2741. This is a national database of products, assistive technology, and rehabilitation equipment available from domestic and international sources.

• **Senior centers provide programs and respite care for primary caregivers.** Especially for family members who need to work outside the home, senior centers have classes, lectures, and outings that are usually free, except for meals. A particular center may be for chronically ill elders who need a place to go for minimal medical care and supervised therapy, as well as socializing.

• **Church and synagogue bulletin boards and newsletters list support organizations and programs for families.** Houses of worship offer spiritual support, as well as community programs.

• **Telephone reassurance and visiting services are helpful and often essential for someone living alone.** Churches, synagogues, hospital auxiliary departments, and volunteer organizations have established telephone projects. Visiting services are offered by a variety of volunteer agencies and organizations, including some labor unions who offer them as benefits to retired members.

• **Transportation services, especially for elderly citizens, are available in many communities.** Cars, buses, and van service, some equipped for disabled passengers and wheelchair users, are provided by various community organizations. Taxi services may offer discounts for senior citizens.

• **Family Service America (FSA) provides family counseling services.** Through its two hundred member agencies nationwide, this organization provides families with information and referral services, as well as counseling and support groups. **FSA is at 11700 West Lake Park Drive, Milwaukee, WI 53224. Call (800) 221-2681 for the agency serving your community.**

• **Adult Day Care Centers provide care for older people who can no longer remain at home alone but who do not need skilled nursing care.** This is a fairly new concept, and centers are not available in all communities. Some facilities are not-for-profit and receive federal and community assistance. Others are privately owned and operated for profit.

• **Geriatric-care managers assist a family member who lives at a distance or who works at a full-time job.** Care managers are social workers, nurses, or psychologists who have private practices to counsel and assist families in planning for long-term care. They arrange for home health care as needed, such as visiting nurses; occupational, physical, speech, or other therapists; and personal-care and homemaker aides. Two national organizations can provide help in locating social workers:

Aging Network Services, Inc., 4400 East-West Hwy., Suite 907, Bethesda, MD 20814, (301) 657-4329, has a national network of 250 geriatric social workers; and the **National Association of Professional Geriatric-Care Managers,** 655 Alvernon Way, Suite 108, Tucson, AZ 85711, (602) 881-8008, sets standards for the profession and acts as a national referral service.

• **Children of Aging Parents, Woodburne Office Campus, Suite 302A, Levittown, PA 19057, (215) 945-6900.** This is a national clearinghouse for caregiving families.

• **Elder Support Network** provides a variety of services based on an ability to pay. With 146 affiliate organizations, this service of the Association of Jewish Family and Children's Agencies has Meals-on-Wheels, respite care, telephone assurance, friendly visiting, home care, and transportation. **Call (800) 677-1116 for an agency in your area.**

Another organization, **Eldercare Locators,** helps callers to find information toll free about community services available throughout the country. They may also be reached at (800) 677-1116.

• **Hospice care is provided in homes.** For information about hospice programs, contact **the National Hospice Organization, 1901 North Moore Street, Suite 901, Arlington, VA 22209, (703) 243-5900.**

• **The Well Spouse Foundation** is a network of support groups for well caregiving spouses. More than seventy-five support groups meet to exchange information among members and support one another. Meetings have invited speakers, discussions, and personal exchanges, and the focus is on the well spouse. The $15 membership fee includes a newsletter. Call or write **Well Spouse Foundation, P.O. Box 801, New York, NY 10023, (212) 724-7209.**

• **American Association of Retired Persons, 601 E**

228 RECOVERING AT HOME AFTER A STROKE

Street, NW, Washington, DC 20049, (202) 434-2277.
This is the world's largest nonprofit, nonpartisan organization dedicated to enhancing the quality of life for older people. The organization offers discounts, free publications, a mail-order pharmacy service, and travel service, to name just a few of their services. The $8 a year membership includes the *AARP News Bulletin* and the magazine *Modern Maturity.*

• **The People's Medical Society is an organization that works to protect medical rights.** For a description of its services, its address and telephone number, see page 42.

SUPPORT GROUPS AND NATIONAL STROKE ASSOCIATIONS

"You get a sense of belonging in a club at a time when you feel like an outsider everywhere else," says a woman who is a member of an aphasia group. "Stroke clubs let you know that there is life after stroke. You go home from a meeting and you realize people are still going about their lives—it's not the end of the world," says another group member. "It's a safe place where you're not being judged. Just when you're feeling rather clumsy, useless, and dependent, it's glorious to know you can help someone else—that gets your juices flowing again."

The names of some stroke clubs reflect the strength of their spirit, as well as their individuality: VALORS (Veteran Assurance League to Obtain Recovery), the Boomerang Club, FOCUS (Families Organized for Community Understanding), OPUS, Inc. (Organization of People Undaunted by Stroke).

The consumer-run groups, organized by men and women who have had a stroke, meet in a place in the community, possibly a church or synagogue, or a senior or community center. They provide a forum for people who have had a stroke to share information and experiences related to living with stroke. Family members, friends, and professionals are welcome to meetings, as well as anyone else who is interested.

Some clubs feature regular weekly daytime activities of crafts, dance therapy, speech and communication groups, discussions, lectures, and social events. Many publish newsletters for their members. The focus may vary from group to group, but all clubs offer members emotional support, practical advice, and a chance to be with people who have had similar experiences.

There are close to nine hundred stroke groups which represent more than 45,000 members in the United States and Canada. Some of the following organizations can direct you to a support group in your community.

• **The American Heart Stroke Connection, 7272 Greenville Avenue, Dallas, TX 75231. You may call (800) 553-6321,** Monday through Friday, 8:30 A.M. to 5:00 P.M., central time, for stroke groups that meet in your community. Many of the groups listed with the Network are associated with local American Heart Association affiliates. They also have groups in several foreign countries.

The Network has excellent training materials for group leaders and groups who want to develop an outreach program to support people who have had a stroke and can benefit from listening to the first-hand experiences of others.

The Network publishes *Stroke Connection*, a newsletter with articles written by consumers who have had a stroke, and information about research from professionals. A subscription is $8. Another publication, *A Stroke of Luck*, is an informal communication newsletter for people with aphasia.

• **National Stroke Association (NSA), 8480 E. Orchard Road, Suite 1000, Englewood, CO 80111-5015, (800) STROKES, (800) 787-6537, or (303) 771-1700.** Founded in 1984, NSA provides nationwide information, education, and referral services for stroke survivors, their families, and health professionals. They offer guidance to people interested in forming stroke clubs and aphasia support groups.

The Association also does outstanding work in reporting the results of professional research, and serves as advocates for stroke survivors. Their quarterly newsletter, *Be Stroke Smart*, is one of the most informative consumer resources available; it includes information on recent medical research, with articles by both professionals and consumers.

Their free or reasonably priced educational materials and audiovisuals include *The Road Ahead: A Stroke Recovery Guide, Disability Work for Social Security Applicants,* and *A Guide to Helping Elderly Relatives Near and Far.* Membership is $10 for anyone concerned about stroke, including stroke survivors and their families, and it includes the newsletter, a 10 percent discount on all NSA materials, and assorted printed materials and audiovisuals.

• **The National Aphasia Association, P.O. Box 1887, Murray Hill Station, New York, NY 10156-0611, (800) 922-4622.** This association is an advocacy group for an estimated one million people who have aphasia. They also can provide information and guidance for people with aphasia and their families.

Heart Support Groups

• **Mended Hearts, 7320 Greenville Avenue, Dallas, TX 75231, (214) 706-7272,** is an organization of 225 chapters run by and for men and women with heart conditions and their families. Meetings feature invited speakers who talk on a variety of health issues, with interactive discussions, rap sessions, and social get-togethers. Annual dues are $15 for individuals, $22 for families; membership includes their newsletter, *Heartbeat*.

• **Coronary Club, Inc., 9500 Euclid Avenue, Cleveland, OH 44195, (216) 444-3690,** with five affiliates, meets to educate and to give mutual support to people with heart conditions and their families. The organization offers a monthly newsletter, *Heartline*, covering a wide range of subjects. A subscription is $29.

FURTHER SUPPORT INFORMATION

• An estimated 15 million people attend weekly **twelvestep support programs**. Another 100 million people—friends and family—encourage them. Groups such as Alcoholics Anonymous, Smokers Anonymous, Overeaters Anonymous, Narcotics Anonymous, and Alanon for family members or friends are listed in your local telephone book.

• **The American Self-Help Clearinghouse, St. Clare's-Riverside Medical Center, Denville, NJ 07834, (201) 625-7101, TDD (201) 625-9053.** Callers on the center's helpline are given information about specific groups of interest to them.

• **The American Chronic Pain Association, P.O. Box 850, Rocklin, CA 95677, (916) 632-9022.** This is a selfhelp organization with over five hundred groups internationally. They offer information and other services to people who have chronic pain and their families.

• **National Handicapped Sports, 451 Hungerford**

Drive, Suite 100, Rockville, MD 20850, (800) 966-4NHS. They give information about sports and recreational activities nationwide for people with disabilities.

• **Help for Incontinent People, Inc. (HIP), P.O. Box 544, Union, SC 29379, (800) 252-3337.** A nonprofit organization, HIP is dedicated to improving the quality of life for people with incontinence. It is a leading source of education and support to the public as well as to health care professionals.

• **Residential Aphasia Program, University of Michigan, Communicative Disorders Clinic, Victor Vaughan Building, 1111 East Catherine Street, Ann Arbor, MI 48109-2054, Voice and TDD (313) 764-8440.** This unique residential aphasia program is offered in six-week sessions throughout the year. It offers many important benefits to stroke survivors including mutual support from peers; opportunities for improving self-help and daily living skills; and the occasion for introspection and priority setting, away from the day-to-day stresses of family life.

SHOPPING FOR USEFUL PRODUCTS

Shopping may be difficult for a number of reasons like: "There isn't enough time in the day." Or, "I simply don't have the energy." "It's too confusing." "There's no transportation I can use to get to the stores."

We asked members of stroke clubs for their recommendations of how to find useful products at reasonable prices. Physical and occupational therapists also were asked for their suggestions of products that provide greater self-sufficiency in everyday living.

Many men and women say that before leaving the hospital, or while in rehabilitation, an occupational therapist recommended utensils or other products they found useful. Some people purchased a few of these items in the hospital. Others decided to wait and see what was available in their local stores or from mail-order catalogs. What they sometimes found was that some products were hard to find or needed to be specially ordered, or were poorly made, unattractive, and overpriced.

"There can be a large price difference for the same item: a bath chair can vary in price as much as $40 in some places," reports a woman who recently had a stroke. "Comparison shopping before making almost any purchase is your only defense. But also consider the quality of the product, the convenience of having the item delivered to your home, and the return policy of the vendor. Most items purchased through mail-order companies are returnable."

Shoppers are encouraged to find stores that carry products they can use. For example:

• **The Home Depot**, a nationwide chain of more than 200 stores, carries a wide selection of items you need to make your bathroom accessible. You can find grab bars, shower and bath chairs, hand-held shower heads, and raised toilet seats.

• **Sears Health Care Catalog, (800) 326-1750,** offers many items including blood pressure monitors, a salt checker which provides a readout of the amount of salt in food, motorized beds, personal-care products, bath chairs, and other practical home-care products.

• **Radio Shack**, another nationwide chain, has reasonably priced intercoms, electronic pill boxes that signal to remind you when to take medication, wireless remote-control devices that will turn on your lights, TV set, and other appliances throughout the house from one central locale.

• **AdaptABILITY** (a division of S & S Worldwide), **(800) 243-9232,** is one of many mail-order companies with products for people with disabilities. They have a large selection of personal-care items, household products, and assistive devices for the activities of daily living. For example, they carry specialized eating utensils, plates, cups, reachers, and easy-jar openers that work with one hand. They also have dressing aids, including a one-hand buttoning and zipping device as well as a gadget that makes putting on socks easier. Call and ask for their catalog to get an idea of their products, their specialties, and to compare prices.

• **Don Krebs' Access to Recreation, (800) 634-4351,** is a catalog offering products for people who enjoy physical activity and have a disability. Some of the equipment that makes this possible are power trainers that can be used from a wheelchair or any sturdy chair, swimming aids that provide support in maintaining a vertical position in the water, and a lightweight aluminum vest and harness that holds a fishing rod to allow you to reel in your catch with one hand. Don Krebs has two other catalogs for consumers of adaptive equipment and generally useful devices for home and office.

• **Bruce Medical Supply, (800) 225-8446,** is another mail-order company that offers a wide range of personal-care products, diabetic accessories and supplies, canes, wheelchairs, and products for incontinence.

• **Avenues Unlimited, Inc., (800) 848-AVES or (800) 848-2837,** is a mail-order division of Everest & Jennings, which sells attractive clothing for the wheelchair user. From basic rain ponchos and jeans to jackets and wool coats, the clothing is designed specifically for maximum comfort while a person is seated. Jackets are cut shorter to stay neat and to clear the wheels, and they have action-back pleats for freedom of arm movement. Hidden wrist loops and longer fly-fronts make dressing easier.

• **Comfortably Yours, (800) 521-0097,** is a mail order company that carries an array of personal-care and household products.

• **Menu Magic, (800) 572-5888,** has introduced pureed entree mixes for people with swallowing difficulties.

• **The American Foundation for the Blind, 15 West 16th Street, New York, NY 10011, (800) 829-0500.** The AFB Product Center's catalog is available in print, Braille, audiocassette, or on diskette. Among the many items they offer are toys and clocks that "talk." Also of particular interest is a Franklin Talking Dictionary, a portable reference with high-quality speech output and a spelling checker; a talking blood-pressure meter, an enlarged insulin syringe support, and a barrel to accept a syringe with magnified numbers for easier reading. They also carry a portable talkman that is specially adapted to play Library of Congress cassettes as well as standard cassettes.

• **National Association for the Visually Handicapped, 22 West 21st Street, New York, NY 10010, (212) 889-3141.** This association has brought together an outstanding catalog of low-vision aids. Among the many items available from them are large-print scores of music and books, calendars, large-type computer software, large-screen television, nonglare television sets, and synthetic speech output devices that allow computer screen information to be read in a synthesized voice. Other attractive products you can't find easily include a talking desk calculator with a big number display; a talking clock that gives the current time in English or Spanish, speaks as you set the time and alarm, and can be set to announce the time on the hour. You may call them to receive a catalog.

• **Home-care stores, surgical-supply companies, and some drugstore chains rent out wheelchairs, motorized beds, and other assistive devices**. Their prices vary considerably for the same type of item. It's a good idea to comparison-shop to get the best price. Some community organizations loan equipment at low cost or free of charge. The selection is not extensive, and you will usually have the responsibility of having it picked up and returned.

• **ABLEDATA, c/o the National Rehabilitation Information Center (NARIC), (800) 346-2741,** is a national database of over 25,000 different adaptive equipment items for daily living, specially designed for people with mobility, visual, communication, and hearing impairments. Among the many materials available from them are legislation pertaining to disability issues, current medical research developments relating to disabilities, and information and resources on financial matters, accessible sports, travel agencies, personal attendants, sexuality, and safety issues. A nominal fee to cover the mailing costs is charged for printed materials.

• *Independent Living*, **150 Motor Parkway, Suite 420, Hauppauge, NY 11788-5145, (516) 273-0066,** is a magazine that is an excellent resource for people with disabilities, connecting them with home health-care dealers and manufacturers by publishing a directory of products and telling where to locate them. It is published seven times a year, and the yearly subscription price is $15.

(If you find products and vendors you think are outstanding, share the information with your therapists and other people you know who have had a stroke who may benefit from your experience.)

SPEECH AND LANGUAGE / INFORMATION AND MATERIALS

Because each person's needs are unique, speech/language ᵇⁿlogists recommend that before you purchase computer software, which is costly, you should ask therapists for their input and recommendations.

• **The Trace Center, S-151 Waisman Center, 1500 Highland Avenue, Madison, WI 53705, (608) 262-6966 and TDD (608) 263-5408,** addresses the communication needs of people who are nonspeaking and have disabilities. They do research in communication and study ways in which people who are nonspeaking and physically disabled can converse and write, including the use of high-technology communication aids.

The Trace Center is an outstanding resource whose communication specialists endeavor to give you support in finding what's appropriate for you among the available computer and communication devices. Seating, positioning, and mobility specialists provide information about communication aids that can be mounted on a wheelchair or carried. They can direct callers to evaluation centers and other community resources.

• **The Speech Bin, (800) 4 SPEECH,** has word-finding and aphasia-rehabilitation workbooks and computer software, some of which you may already have used in speech therapy and in aphasia groups. Call for their catalog and discuss with your therapist which items are best for you.

• **Imaginart Communication Products, (800) 828-1376,** has speech, language, and learning materials for stroke survivors and their families. One item that is useful, for example, is an augmentative communication system that works with stickers. They carry photo cards, workbooks, flash cards, and a word finder. They also offer food-thickening agents to provide safe swallowing.

• **Wayne State University Press, the Leonard N. Simons Building, 5959 Woodward Avenue, Detroit, MI 48202, (313) 577-6120** is another good resource for communication-skills materials.

• **Toward Independence** is a catalog offered by the

Attainment Company, Inc., (800) 327-4269. They offer step-by-step illustrated cards and guides for shopping, cooking, community activities, grooming, and housekeeping. Life-skill and work-activity materials for communicating, sequencing, and time managing are available. Many men and women find that books of regular and enlarged-type word finders, as well as workbooks with lessons in writing, reading, and arithmetic, are useful in reintroducing language. Some people enjoy talking books, as well as Scrabble, Monopoly, Bingo, and similar games.

COMPUTERS / INFORMATION AND SOFTWARE

Many men and women find the computer to be an invaluable tool in restoring communication skills. "You can work independently with software," says a man who before his stroke didn't use a computer. "You eliminate the middleman of someone who is teaching you with flash cards; it's just you and the computer talking to one another."

If you have a computer, or access to one, you may want to obtain software to help you hone your communication skills. It is wise to consult your therapist for program recommendations.

• **SeniorNet, (415) 750-5030,** is a nonprofit membership organization for people fifty-five and over who presently use a computer or would like to learn. Located in a variety of facilities—such as senior community centers and schools and college campuses—their Learning Centers are sponsored by local organizations and offer classes that are budget priced. Call SeniorNet to find out if there is a Learning Center near you.

• **Parrot Software, 190 Sandy Ridge Road, State College, PA 16803, (800) PARROT-1 or (814) 237-7282,** works primarily with speech and language pathologists but will give you and your therapist information about their software programs for people with aphasia and other communication problems. The Parrot "Peace of Mind Policy" offers personal attention to all software questions, a consultation with a computer-knowledgeable speech pathologist who will help you select the best software for your needs, plus a free thirty-day trial.

• **Creative Learning, 206 Sacramento Street, Suite 305, Nevada City, CA 95959, (916) 265-0584,** offers an award-winning computer software series for people who have had a stroke. It includes picture commands, the human voice, and touch windows to teach basic language skills.

TELEPHONES AND OTHER COMMUNICATION AIDS

• **The AT&T Accessible Communication Products Center, (800) 233-1222,** offers products designed to enhance the day-to-day communications of people who have disabilities. Call between 8:30 A.M. and 6:30 P.M., eastern time, for information about their telephones with hearing amplification, large-button dials, text telephones or (TDD), automatic dialing, and hands-free speaker phones that let you place or receive telephone calls independently.

• **Telephone companies have an operator-supported service that will type a message to a TDD from a voice caller.**

• **Many stores like Radio Shack carry phones with**

amplification, speaker phones, and large-button telephones.

• **AdaptABILITY** carries a gooseneck shaft with clamp that securely fastens to most surfaces and holds any receiver in a stationary, accessible position. Call them at **(800) 243-9232.**

• **Sears Health Care Catalog, (800) 326-1750,** has a phone with memory dialing combined with a personal emergency response system. At the touch of a button—on the phone or a pendant remote control—preprogrammed emergency numbers are dialed and a clear, concise message and request for assistance are transmitted. The telephone is operated by touching the large, illuminated keypad or by pressing the button on the remote pendant.

Close-Captioned Televisions and Decoders

All television sets now manufactured must have the capacity to access captioning. Ultimately, all programs will have captions.

• The original target audience for captioning was thirteen million people who are hearing impaired, but the audience is considerably larger today as an increasing number of people find support in seeing the written word while it is being spoken. **The National Captioning Institute (NCI), 5203 Leesburg Pike, Suite 1500, Falls Church, VA 22041, (703) 998-2400,** has information about the features and benefits of captioning. The Institute repairs all decoders, no matter where they were purchased.

• **Sears, Circuit City, and Service Merchandise carry telecaption decoders by NCI** which, when hooked up to an existing television, VCR, cable converter, or satellite receiver, will use the remote control from one of these devices to change channels.

Free Loan Service of Open-Captioned Films

• **Modern Talking Picture Service, 5000 Park Street North, St. Petersburg, FL 33709, (800) 237-6213,** is a free loan service of open-captioned films and videos that are available to hearing-impaired individuals, as well as other people who would benefit from seeing captions, and to organizations. More than 3,000 films and videos include ˙ entertainment, adult-educational, and special-interest categories.

Free Radio Reading Services

• **The National Association of Radio Reading Services, 2100 Wharton Street, Suite 140, Pittsburgh, PA 15203, (412) 488-3944.** Many of the nation's leading newspapers and magazines are read over the airwaves by a full-time radio reading service. For people who would benefit from this service and qualify, free radios carrying the special station are provided. Call the association to locate the reading service in your area.

BOOKS

The following list contains only a few of the outstanding books available on the subject of stroke and related topics. Included are books on home nursing care, diet, medications, and exercise, as well as heart conditions, high blood pressure, and diabetes.

About Stroke

DONNAN, GEOFFREY, AND CAROL BURTON
After a Stroke: A Support Book for Patients, Caregivers, Families and Friends
North Atlantic Books, 1990
   Contributing rehabilitation specialists of the Australian Brain Foundation's Stroke Assistance Service blend traditional medicine with movement therapies and body work to stimulate and reeducate the brain and neural-limb coordination.

EWING, SUSAN ADAIR AND BETH PFALZGRAF
Pathways: Moving Beyond Stroke and Aphasia
National Stroke Association
   An intimate description of the experiences of six individuals and their families as stroke and aphasia invade their lives. In addition to being profoundly moving, the book provides a profile of issues that are universal to anyone who has had a stroke, and their family. The book and two outstanding accompanying videotapes of *Pathways* are available from the National Stroke Association at (800) STROKES.

GORDON, NEIL
Stroke: Complete Exercise Guide
Human Kinetics, 1993
   A comprehensive step-by-step guide to safe exercise for stroke survivors.

KASELL, PAT AND HEDDA SCHLOSBERG
The One-Handed Way: Living with the Use of One Hand
American Heart Stroke Connection, 1993

Here are new ways to accomplish daily routines with easy-to-follow directions and picture guides. Some topics covered include kitchen tips, getting dressed, laundry, personal care, and leisure activities. Available from the American Heart Association's Stroke Connection Network at (800) 553-6321.

The Road Ahead
National Stroke Association
This useful guide for stroke survivors and their families is intended to answer many of the questions that arise during recovery from a stroke. Topics include common concerns of caregivers, goal-setting procedures and progress log sheet, sexuality, and changing relationships. There are also clear explanations pertaining to communication, cognition, and visual problems. Available from the National Stroke Association at (800) STROKES.

Home Nursing Care

ZASTOCKI, DEBORAH K., AND CHRISTINE A. ROVINSKI
Home Care: Patient and Family Instructions
W. B. Saunders Company, 1989
A collection of ready-to-use self-care instructions tailored for families to use at home. In clear and simple nontechnical language, the book covers what you will want to know about home nursing care.

Caring

FOYER, JOAN ELLEN
Family Caregiver's Guide
National Stroke Association
This how-to book not only explains how to care for a loved one but also presents a practical approach based on the

simple theory that the caregiver who is strong, happy, and efficient will be far more useful than one who is overwhelmed by emotional pressures, exhausted by inefficient work methods, and resentful of the responsibilities.

Take Care!
Wilder Foundation
A thirty-page booklet, *Take Care!* is a quick and encouraging self-care course for caregivers. It gives specific suggestions leading toward an understanding of some sources of stress and advice on how to set realistic expectations and limits. To order, send $2.50 to Community Care Resources, the Amherst H. Wilder Foundation, *Take Care!*, 919 Lafond Avenue, St. Paul, MN 55104.

Incontinence

BURGIO, KATHRYN L., K. LYNETTE PEARCE, AND ANGELO J. LUCCO
Staying Dry: A Practical Guide to Bladder Control
Johns Hopkins, 1989
Based on a program developed by the National Institute on Aging, the book combines medical advice with a step-by-step supportive plan.

Medications

About Your High Blood Pressure Medicines
U.S. Pharmacopoeial Convention (USP)
This $7.50 paperback includes an easy-to-understand explanation of high blood pressure and the drugs used for its treatment.

About Your Medicines
U.S. Pharmacopoeial Convention (USP)

This $7.95 paperback is a consumer guide to the most commonly used prescription drugs and includes discussions of a medicine's proper use, side effects, and precautions about drug and food interactions. It contains both a brand- and generic-name index.

DR. H. WINTER GRIFFIN
The Complete Guide to Prescription and Non-Prescription Drugs
The Body Press/Perigee, 1992
This paperback provides information on 5,000 brand names and generic drugs in easy-to-read charts. Each chart includes the dosage and usage, possible adverse reactions or side effects, symptoms of overdose, warnings and precautions, and possible interaction with other drugs, food, and other substances.

Well-being

BENSON, HERBERT, AND ELLEN M. STUART, AND THE STAFF OF THE MIND/BODY MEDICAL INSTITUTE
The Wellness Book: The Comprehensive Guide to Maintaining Health and Treating Stress-Related Illness
Fireside/Simon and Schuster, 1993
A workbook following the program of the Mind/Body Medical Institute, it includes stress management, exercise, and nutrition, to provide a complete guide for enhancing health and dealing with cardiovascular and most other illnesses. For audiotapes of the program, see page 252.

BURNS, DAVID D.
The Feeling Good Handbook: Using the New Mood Therapy in Everyday Life
William Morrow, 1989
The author of *Feeling Good*, a best-seller on depression, now shows you how to develop self-esteem, enjoy greater intimacy, and overcome anxiety, fears, and phobias.

COPELAND, MARY ELLEN
The Depression Workbook
New Harbinger, 1992
   Here is self-help guidance for using relaxation, diet, exercise, and full-spectrum light to stabilize moods and increase self-confidence and self-esteem. It also offers
   suggestions for finding high-quality professionals.

MOHS-CATALANO, ELLEN M.
Chronic Pain Control Work Book
New Harbinger, 1987
   This book helps provide understanding of various types of
   pain, as well as offering specific home strategies to reduce
   pain and cope with discomfort.

SELIGMAN, MARTIN E. P.
Learned Optimism
Pocket, 1990
   This guide outlines easy-to-follow techniques that have
   helped thousands of people rise above pessimism and the
   depression that accompanies negative thoughts.

SOTILE, WAYNE M.
*Intimacy and Heart Illness: How Caring Relationships Aid Re-
covery*
Johns Hopkins, 1992
   This is a reassuring consumer's guide to the common concerns about sex and intimacy and heart illness. See the
   audiovisuals on page 252 for more about Dr. Sotile's program.

TUBESING, DONALD A.
Kicking Your Stress Habits
Whole Person Associates, Inc., 1981
   Here is a workbook that helps you identify your beliefs,
   values, and goals in order to focus on what really matters

and, in so doing, worry less about irrelevant events or concerns. To order, call or write Whole Person Associates, P.O. Box 3151, Duluth, MN 55803, (218) 727-0500.

YAPKO, MICHAEL D.
Free Yourself from Depression
Rodale, 1992
   This is a step-by-step exploration of causes of depression and ways to reclaim self-esteem, silence your inner critic, and stand by yourself.

Heart

DEBAKEY, MICHAEL E., AND ANTONIO M. GROTTO, JR., LYNN W. SCOTT, AND JOHN P. FOREYT
The Living Heart: Brand Name Shopper's Guide
Master Media, 1992
   Take Dr. DeBakey's book along on your next shopping trip. It's a guide to thousands of brand-name products that are low in fat and have the blessings of a renowned cardiac surgeon.

LEGATO, MARIANNE J., AND CAROL COLEMAN
The Female Heart: The Truth about Women and Coronary Heart Disease
Simon & Schuster, 1991
   This book replaces the myth that heart disease is only a man's problem with vital information.

ORNISH, DEAN
Dr. Dean Ornish's Program for Reversing Heart Disease
Ballantine, 1992
   Topics covered in this book include managing stress through meditation, psychological counseling, and peer support, with guidelines for diet and exercise. You will find

excellent low-fat heart-healthy meals. See the audiovisuals
section on page 253 for more about Dr. Ornish's program.

PISCATELLA, JOSEPH
Controlling Your Fat Tooth
Workman, 1991
> The author of *Don't Eat Your Heart Out Cookbook* and
> *Choices for a Healthy Heart* creates a simple do-it-yourself
> approach to managing fat in your diet without feeling
> deprived.

PRITIKIN, ROBERT
The New Pritikin Program
Pocket, 1991
> Here is the Pritikin eating plan and pioneering lifestyle
> approach to controlling and reversing most heart condi-
> tions. See the list of newsletters on page 250 for more
> information about Pritikin programs.

Diabetes

BIERMANN, JUNE, AND BARBARA TOOKEY
The Diabetic's Book: All Your Questions Answered
Tarcher/Perigee, 1992
> Here are clear and comprehensive answers to the most
> commonly asked questions about diabetes by the founders
> and directors of the Sugar Free Center, a national mail-
> order source of diabetes information and products.

EDELWICH, JERRY, AND ARCHIE BRODSKY
Caring for Your Emotions as Well as Your Health
Chronimed, 1992
> This book is more than a manual on testing blood and
> taking insulin shots; the authors draw upon their firsthand
> knowledge of living with diabetes to share their valuable
> wisdom and experience with the reader.

Eliminating Physical- and Emotional-Risk Factors

FERGUSON, TOM
*The No-Nag, No-Guilt, Do-It-Your-Own-Way Guide to
Quitting Smoking*
Ballantine, 1987
   Here are the steps to take toward becoming a permanent
   nonsmoker, plus information for families and friends who
   want to support the effort. See the audiovisuals section on
   page 252 for information about helping someone get ready
   to quit smoking.

LIEBELT, ROBERT
Straight Talk About Alcoholism
Pharos Books, 1992
   A doctor explains the causes of alcoholism, its effects, and
   what you can do about it.

WILLIAMS, REDFORD
The Trusting Heart: Great News About Type A Behavior
Times Books/Random House, 1989
   A detailed review of the research showing that hostility is
   the only unhealthy component of Type A behavior.

WILLIAMS, REDFORD, AND VIRGINIA WILLIAMS
*Anger Kills: Seventeen Strategies for Reducing the Hostility That
Can Harm Your Health*
Times Books/Random House, 1992
   How to tell if you have a hostile personality, its affect on
   your heart, and what to do about it if you do.

NEWSLETTERS

Travelin' Talk. A quarterly newsletter that has news, tips,
and resources from a membership network of people as-

sisting travelers with disabilities. The one-time registration fee is on a sliding scale. A 500-page member directory of resources is available for $35. It includes listings of the members of the network, the information they share, and the services they provide; it also comes complete with road maps. Call or write *Travelin' Talk*, P.O. Box 3534, Clarksville, TN 37043-3334, (615) 552-6670.

Tufts University Diet & Nutrition Letter (monthly) from Tufts, P.O. Box 5787, Boulder, CO 89322-7857, (800) 274-7581.

Harvard Heart Letter (monthly) from Harvard Heart Letter, P.O. Box 420234, Palm Coast, FL 32142-0234.

University of California Berkeley Wellness Letter (monthly) from University of California, Berkeley Wellness Letter, P.O. Box 359148, Palm Coast, FL 32035.

Pritikin Vantage Point (monthly) from Pritikin Systems, Inc., 1910 Ocean Front Walk, Santa Monica, CA 90405. To learn about the Pritikin Longevity Centers and their programs call (800) 421-9911.

Food News for Consumers (4 issues per year), published by the USDA Food Safety and Inspection Service. Order from the Superintendent of Documents, U.S. Government Printing Office, Washington, DC 20402. For a listing of "Publications for Sale," contact Human Nutrition Information Service, USDA, 6505 Belcrest Road, Hyattsville, MD 20782; (301) 436-8498.

AUDIOVISUALS

American Heart Stroke Connection
Stroke Survivor's Workout is a 28 minute video of exercises that can be done from a standard chair or wheelchair, and others that can be done while standing and using a chair for support. The video costs $6, and includes the shipping. Call (800) 553-6321.

National Stroke Association
Pathways is the compelling, true-life account of six people who struggle through and overcome—each in his or her unique way—the aftermath of stroke and aphasia in their everyday lives. *What Is Aphasia?* revisits the same six participants of *Pathways* and gives an in-depth explanation of aphasia and its differences in each individual. These two videotapes are available from the National Stroke Association at (800) STROKES.

Occu-Ther, Inc., Productions
Stroke-A-Cize is a guided arm-and-leg mobility exercise program involving the sound side and mobilizing the weaker. Developed by an occupational therapist, the exercises are performed while seated. Available from Occu-Ther, Inc., Productions, 11316 Lakeshore Drive West, Carmel, IN 46032.

Senior Fitnessize
Available in both audio and videotape formats with accompanying manual, this will assist you in range-of-motion and muscle-toning exercises while seated. Available from *Senior Fitnessize*, P.O. Box 2567, Morganton, North Carolina 28655, (704) 438-9274; they will send you a free brochure.

Swing into Shape
These low-intensity nonaerobic videotapes come in 3 different levels. Level 1 is 30 minutes long, and done while seated; levels 2 and 3 are more intensive. Available from the **Swing into Shape** catalog, the Product Marketing Line of the Lutheran Hospital, Department of Education, 1910 South Avenue, La Cross, WI 54601, (608) 791-4787.

Cardiac Couples
The Couple's Journey: The Challenge of Change in Marriage; Sex, Intimacy and Health; Thriving, Not Just Surviving all are audiotapes by Dr. Wayne M. Sotile, author of *Heart Illness and Intimacy*. Available from Cardiac Couples, c/o Wayne M. Sotile, 1396 Old Mill Circle, Winston-Salem, NC 27103, (919) 765-3032.

Self-Care Productions
Helping Smokers Get Ready to Quit is a book and audiotape program written by Dr. Tom Ferguson, author of *The No-Nag, No-Guilt, Do-It-Your-Own-Way Guide to Quitting Smoking*. Available from Great Performance, 14964 NW Greenbrier Pkwy., Beaverton, OR 97006-5797, (800) 433-3803.

The Mind/Body Medical Institute
Relaxation response audiotapes used in their program for people dealing with cardiac rehabilitation, hypertension, pain, and other stress-related medical conditions are available from The Mind/Body Medical Institute, Division of Behavioral Medicine, New England Deaconess Hospital, 185 Pilgrim Road, Boston, MA 02215, (617) 632-9530.

Mind/Body Health Sciences, Inc.
Guided meditation and relaxation audiotapes designed to promote inner wisdom and healing, as well as a

quarterly newsletter that gives information about workshops and trainings by Joan and Myroslav Borysenko, are available from Mind/Body Health Sciences, Inc., 393 Dixon Road, Salina Route, Boulder, CO 80302, (303) 440-8460.

Stress-Reduction Tapes

Mindfulness meditation practice tapes led by Jon Zabet Zinn are used at the University of Massachusetts Medical Center's Stress Reduction Clinic. The audiotapes are available from Stress Reduction Tapes, P.O. Box 547, Lexington, MA 02173.

Dr. Dean Ornish's Program

Audiotapes of *Dr. Dean Ornish's Program for Reversing Heart Disease*, which embodies a mind-body approach to recovery, and of *Eat More, Weigh Less* are available in bookstores.

Peaceful Warrior Services

When the Going Gets Tough, Rules for Being Human, The Peaceful Warrior are among the audiotapes offered to expand awareness, inspire action, and uplift the spirit. Available from Peaceful Warrior Services, P.O. Box 6148-Dept. NOM, San Rafael, CA 94903, (415) 491-0301.

ANN FARRONE*, A CHEF

I had my stroke right before I was going into the hospital for a heart valve replacement operation. I was in the doctor's office getting my blood tested and I had an EKG, and that's when I had the stroke. I was taken from there directly to a local hospital. After that, I went into a rehabilitation center.

The stroke affected my right side, and it's still not right. Once in a while, I still walk crooked, like when I'm very tired. And my right shoulder is not yet one hundred percent, so I do a lot of things with my left hand. At first, I couldn't talk very well, so I had speech therapy at home for about two months. Then when I felt better and was able to go out, I went to a facility at my local hospital twice a week for therapy. Once every third week they would have a group session for speech therapy. I did that for a long time and it did help.

I live with my husband, and it's just the two of us at home now. This experience has taken its toll on him. He came to see me every day while I was in the hospital, and that's quite a trip from here. Then I came home from the hospital, and he did everything. And there was a lot of crying then. I cried when my husband *did* do something. I cried when he *didn't* do something the way *I* would have done it. And when he saw that I was crying, he would be upset and say, "Ann, are you crying again?" Well, one day my friend said to me, "You have every reason to cry." This way of putting it made me feel better because she didn't talk against my husband, and she even acknowledged that she understood he had been through a lot himself. She just indicated that I was entitled to my feelings, and she made me feel better.

* This is a pseudonym.

My friends have helped me an awful lot. When they came to see me after I got home from the hospital, they took me anyplace I wanted to go. And when they came, they would tell me how much better I sounded. That made a big difference in my life—gave me a lot of encouragement and hope. I had been worried that they'd jump in and say words for me when words were difficult for me to find. But most of my friends were patient and waited until I got it myself.

> "If you give yourself a chance, and participate in everything and do everything you can, you do get better."

You have to have faith and you have to persevere, no matter how much you cry or hurt. If you have trouble doing something, don't give up—just go back and do it again. I have my faith in God, and my prayers. If you give yourself a chance, and participate in everything and do everything you can, you do get better.

Afterword

If you have been using this book, you have made the transition from the hospital to your home. Chances are that you have steadily regained your strength and recuperated in various ways. Possibly, you've done this with the help of your family and learned when and how to call on them for help. You've taken charge of your health with the guidance of your doctors and other professionals. You've learned to set your personal goals, monitor your diet and exercise, stopped smoking, and become aware of the cause of daily stress and how to use relaxation techniques to control it. You probably have developed many strategies of your own to make life work for you.

All the lifestyle modifications that are recommended for you are actually no different from what doctors prescribe for people who want to *prevent* stroke. In fact, the healthy choices that you are making can influence family members and friends to take a good, hard look at their own health habits, diet, exercise, and stress-reduction techniques (if any). If this book has helped you to improve the quality of your own life and the lives of people close to you, it will have served its purpose well.

Your experiences can positively influence many people if you share what you have learned as a result of your stroke. For example, you may be able to save someone's life by telling coworkers, neighbors, and others about the warning signs of a stroke. A person who experiences any of these symptoms should not merely wait for them to subside but must get immediate medical care.

Probably the most important sharing you will do will be with people who have just had a stroke. You may want to become a volunteer worker at a hospital, rehabilitation center, or a center for older people or for people with disabilities. Your advice can be more influential than the recommendations of professionals.

At this particular time, you probably are not ready to help other people. When you are, you will experience a life-affirming sense of strength and gratification. This then will be the greatest reward to you and to the authors of this book.

About the Authors

Florence Weiner has written several books about survival and disability, including *No Apologies: A Guide to Living with a Disability*, *Help for the Handicapped Child* and *How to Survive in New York with Children*. She is a disability rights activist and cofounder with Harriet Bell of the Polio Information Center.

Mathew H. M. Lee, M.D., F.A.C.P., has been a rehabilitation physician for thirty-five years and is currently Medical Director at the Rusk Institute of Rehabilitation Medicine, New York University Medical Center, in New York City. He is also Professor, Clinical Rehabilitation Medicine, and Clinical Professor, Behavioral Sciences and Community Health at New York University. Dr. Lee is the editor of *Rehabilitation, Music and Human Well-Being*.

Harriet Bell, Ph.D., was formerly a member of the New York State Board for Nursing, past president of the Auxiliary, and the Community Board at Goldwater Memorial Hospital, Roosevelt Island, New York, where she lived for twenty-five years after contracting polio. Dr. Bell now lives in the community.

Numbers to Call in an Emergency

(in LARGE, BOLD print, write the name and the number of the people you need to call in an emergency)

NAME (Your Doctor):

TELEPHONE NO.:

NAME (Emergency Medical Service):

TELEPHONE NO.:

NAME (Hospital):

TELEPHONE NO.:

NAME (Family Member at Work):

TELEPHONE NO.:

NAME:

TELEPHONE NO.:

NAME:

TELEPHONE NO.:

NAME:

TELEPHONE NO.:

Notes

Notes

Index